HANDBOOK OF

Geriatric Psychopharmacology

Michael A. Jenike

PSG PUBLISHING COMPANY, INC.
LITTLETON, MASSACHUSETTS

Library of Congress Cataloging in Publication Data
Jenike, Michael A.
    Handbook of geriatric psychopharmacology.

    Includes index.
    1. Geriatric psychiatry—Handbooks, manuals, etc. 2. Psychopharmacology—
Handbooks, manuals, etc. I. Title. [DNLM: 1. Mental Disorders—drug therapy. 2. Mental
Disorders—in old age. 3. Psychopharmacology—in old age. WT 150 J51h]
RC451.4.A5J44   1985   618.97'689'18   85-3580
ISBN 0-88416-520-5

Published by:
PSG PUBLISHING COMPANY, INC.
545 Great Road
Littleton, Massachusetts 01460

Printed in the United States of America.

International Standard Book Number: 0-88416-520-5

Library of Congress Catalog Card Number: 85-3580

Last digit is the print number: 9 8 7 6 5 4 3 2

To Nancy, Lisa, Eric, Sara, Una, Andrew, and Ian with love.

ABOUT THE AUTHOR

Michael A. Jenike, M.D. is Director of the Inpatient Psychiatric Service at Massachusetts General Hospital and Assistant Professor of Psychiatry at Harvard Medical School. In addition, he is the Co-Director of the Geriatric Psychiatry Memory Disorders Clinic and Director of the Obsessive-Compulsive Disorders Clinic.

A psychiatrist with extensive experience in clinical geriatric psychopharmacology, Dr. Jenike has conducted a number of research studies in clinical psychopharmacology and has published over 50 scientific and clinical papers. He is the editor of the monthly newsletter, *Massachusetts General Hospital Topics in Geriatrics*, and is co-editor of the psychiatry section of *Scientific American Medicine*. He is a member of a number of professional societies including the American Geriatrics Society, the Gerontological Society of America, the American Psychiatric Association, the American Medical Association, and the Academy of Psychosomatic Medicine.

Dr. Jenike has lectured nationally to physicians and mental health professionals on the topics of geriatric psychopharmacology and Alzheimer's disease and has conducted a number of symposia on the drug treatment of psychiatric illness.

CONTENTS

FOREWORD

"How old would you be if you didn't know how old you were?" asked Satchel Page. That is a good question. Aging is defined in various ways, only one of which depends upon the number of years spent on this earth. George Bernard Shaw, Bernard Baruch, and Pablo Picasso were in their full power of adulthood as septuagenarians. Henry VIII of Great Britain, Louis XII of France, and Maximillian of Germany—all contemporaries whose reigns were marked by change and vigorous rule—became old men by their own and others' accounts, in their mid 50s. Insomnia, spells of melancholia, failing mental powers, and somatic preoccupation besieged these dynastic sovereigns, and each felt the chill shadow of old age. The toll of symptoms and the sense of aging mark an individual's progress along time's course perhaps as accurately as the kitchen calendar.

It is the rare practicing M.D. who is not called upon to deal with one of the conspicuous mental problems of aging. Royalty has no lien on depression, troubled sleep, fading memory, or hypochondriasis. Add anxiety, neurasthenia, chronic pain, and emotional lability, and the series becomes a checklist of the most common maladies found in a psychogeriatric clinic. These very real disorders are as much a part of aging as are the varying grades of renal, pulmonary, hepatic, and cardiac impairment that plague the human organism as it lives out its allotment of years. Because aging so often entails discomfort as well as inefficiency, it is no wonder that older persons seek relief more frequently and more diligently than the young.

I can remember my great aunt, a dourly anergic widow who regularly visited a downtown health parlor in Cincinnati, Ohio, for high colonic irrigations. She got these awesome infusions whenever she suffered her "spells." I don't know what name to give her condition, but I do recall that her spirits improved mightily after this purging. She took this cure well into her 80th year. She also took a variety of other nostrums dispensed by our family doctor, none of which did the job as well as the enema. Our physician was strongly opposed to these colonic infusions, but had nothing in his pharmacopea to match them.

Such is not the case today. I suspect my aunt had chronic constipation, a common geriatric ailment, but linked to this symptom was melancholia, easy fatigue, anxiety, and loneliness, all of which made her feel ancient and useless. At the risk of perforating her bowel, she endured the discomfort of an internal lavage to clear out—as she saw it — the detritus of advancing years. I could be mistaken. For all I know she may have displaced her sexuality to her sigmoid flexure and gotten a libidinal charge from the visit, but I doubt it. Were she alive today I think her trouble might be helped with an antidepressant. I would, in any event, refer her to Dr. Jenike.

As Dr. Jenike clearly outlines, we have a variety of effective pharmaceutical agents for many of the symptoms and disorders of the geriatric population. Dispensing these drugs to elderly persons, however, requires as much specialized skill as does pediatric psychopharmacology. Without doubt, over the course of time geriatric psychopharmacology will be rightfully acknowledged as a medical subspecialty. As our aging population expands and its demands for better mental health grow apace, there will be a greater call for safe and effective psychopharmaceuticals to ward off depression, amnesia, anxiety, insomnia and the other horsemen of the apocalypse of aging. Sagacious, experienced, and judicious clinicians like Dr. Jenike will be turned to for guidance in the selection and use of such pharmaceuticals. This book will be an important medical reference.

Thomas P. Hackett, M.D.
Chief of Psychiatry
Massachusetts General Hospital

PREFACE

Over the last few years the field of geriatrics has grown immensely. As the absolute number of elderly people grows in the United States, the need for physicians to acquire a specialized body of knowledge becomes more pronounced.

This book has been prepared to address directly some of the difficult treatment decisions which face the primary care physician. Physicians of all disciplines come into contact with elderly patients who may be depressed, demented, anxious, or psychotic. Insomnia and the sequellae of toxic drug interactions are frequently encountered.

Handbook of Geriatric Psychopharmacology is an attempt to recommend specific medications for particular situations in order to maximize therapeutic benefits and minimize unwanted side effects.

I wish to express my sincere thanks to my secretary, Nancy Regan, whose dedicated efforts are greatly appreciated.

Michael A. Jenike, M.D.

"Aging is when your little black book contains only names ending in M.D."

CHAPTER 1

Introduction

EMPATHY

The following poem was found among the personal possessions of an elderly woman who had died in a nursing home in Scotland. All of us who deal with the elderly should refer to it from time to time.

A Crabbit Old Woman Wrote This

What do you see, nurses, what do you see?
Are you thinking when you look at me —
A crabbit old woman, not very wise,
Uncertain of health, with far-away eyes,
Who dribbles her food and makes no reply
When you say in a loud voice,
"I do wish you'd try."
Who seems not to notice the things that you do,
And forever is losing a stocking or shoe.
Who unresisting or not, lets you do as you will,
With bathing and feeding, the long day to fill.
Is that what you're thinking,
    is that what you see?
Then open your eyes, nurse,
    you're not looking at me.
I'll tell you who I am as I sit here so still,
As I rise at your bidding, as I eat at your will.
I'm a small child of ten with a father and mother,
Brothers and sisters, who love one another;
A young girl of sixteen with wings on her feet,
Dreaming that soon now a lover I'll meet;
A bride soon at twenty — my heart gives a leap,

1

Remembering the vows that I promised to keep;
At twenty-five now I have young of my own,
Who need me to build a secure happy home:
A woman of thirty, my young now grow fast,
Bound to each other with ties that should last;
At forty, my young sons have grown and are gone,
But my man's beside me to see I don't mourn;
At fifty once more babies play round my knee,
Again we know children, my loved one and me.
Dark days are upon me, my husband is dead,
I look at the future, I shudder with dread.
For my young are all rearing young of their own.
And I think of the years and
    the love that I've known.
I'm an old woman now and nature is cruel —
'Tis her jest to make old age look like a fool.
The body is crumbled, grace and vigor depart,
There now is a stone where I once had a heart.
But inside this old carcass a young girl still dwells,
And now and again my battered heart swells.
I remember the years, I remember the pain,
And I'm loving and living life over again.
I think of the years all too few — gone too fast,
And accept the stark fact that nothing can last.
So open your eyes, nurses, open and see
Not a crabbit old woman, look close — see ME.

DEMOGRAPHY AND GOALS

More than 25 million Americans are over the age of 65 years, roughly 11% of the United States population. It is estimated that by the year 2030, nearly 52 million people — 17% of the population — will exceed age 65. Presently, those over age 65 spend about one fourth of the national total for medication (Vestal, 1984). As we all know far too well, the elderly suffer from many concurrent acute and chronic diseases. In one study of 200 consecutively admitted patients, 78% had at least four major diseases, 38% had six or more, and 13% had eight or more (Wilson et al, 1962). The elderly are clearly more susceptible to disease and are also more vulnerable to side effects from the medications used to treat these illnesses. Fewer than 5% of this group abstain from all drug use (Guttmann, 1978).

Superimposed upon these physical ailments, mental illness in the elderly is common. A recent National Institute of Mental Health (NIMH) study, looking at approximately 10,000 people aged 18 years and older, found that about 19% of the United States population — approximately 29 million people — are suffering from a mental illness (*Psychiatric News,* 1984). Depression is common, with depressive symptoms reported in as many as 20% of healthy adults (Busse, 1978). Alzheimer's disease is now felt to be present in 5% to 7% of those over age 65, and in 20% of those over age 80. Over 10 billion of the 21 billion dollars spent on nursing care in the United States in 1982 was expended on the care of patients with dementing illness and about half of all nursing home beds are occupied by Alzheimer's victims. Many dementing patients suffer from superimposed treatable symptoms such as depression, agitation, confusion, and/or psychosis.

Anxiety disorders are extremely common in the elderly and in the NIMH study were found to be the most common psychiatric disorders in the United States. Sleep disorders occur as a primary disorder or may accompany anxiety, depression, or dementia. In one large survey, 40% of subjects over age 50 complained of insomnia (Bixler et al, 1979).

Because of the prevalence of psychiatric disorders and symptoms in the elderly, every practicing clinician is confronted with these complicated situations. Psychotropic drugs are now among the most frequently prescribed agents in the aged (Greenblatt et al, 1975; Parry et al, 1973; Vestal, 1984). Unfortunately, many of these drugs have side effects, and considerable clinical skill and knowledge is required in order to maximize effectiveness and minimize unwanted effects (Salzman, 1984). Side effects can also be used therapeutically. For instance, a depressed patient with pronounced secondary sleeplessness will benefit much from a sedating antidepressant given near bedtime.

The elderly are not only more sensitive to the adverse effects of the psychotropic agents, but also exhibit an increased variability of response to these drugs. Interindividual differences are much more pronounced in the elderly than they are in the young. Many elderly patients will need similar doses of medication as younger patients. On the other hand, others may need one tenth the dosage.

This book will present an approach to the elderly patient with psychiatric symptoms which will allow the clinician to optimally manage the elderly patient in order to maximize benefit and minimize unwanted effects.

MENTAL STATUS EXAMINATION

Before psychotropic medication is begun, it is essential that the patient's illness be correctly diagnosed. Successful treatment depends to a major extent on the adequacy of the initial evaluation of social and psychological functioning. Pfeiffer has noted that while the *diagnosis* may be based largely on the presence of specific *psychological symptoms,* the *prognosis* will depend heavily on the *social context* in which those psychological symptoms exist (Pfeiffer, 1980).

It is essential to get a past psychiatric history of the elderly patient; it is often necessary to question family members. The patient's previous level of functioning, as well as coping styles, require careful assessment. For instance, if one is called to evaluate a hospitalized patient for dementia and it turns out that one week ago he was working and functioning well, it is likely that the patient is delirious and not demented and treatable causes become the main focus of attention rather than chronic management.

A number of questions can be helpful in assessing base-line social functioning. Does the patient live alone? Does she have friends? Does he belong to any social organizations? Is he married?

Before psychotropic medication is begun, it is necessary to decide who will be following and who, if anyone, will be supervising doses.

Each elderly patient should be questioned in reference to symptoms of depression, anxiety, psychosis, and cognitive dysfunction.

Several tests of cognition are available but are time-consuming and require some expertise to interpret (Jenike, 1982). Two tests that are easily performed and are valid detectors of organic brain disease in the elderly are the Set Test and the Mini-Mental State Exam. A score below 15 on the Set Test or below 12 on the Mini-Mental State Exam correlates with dementia and necessitates a thorough medical workup (see chapter 6).

Set Test: The Set Test was developed in 1972 as a specific screening test for dementia in the elderly (Isaacs and Kennie, 1973). The test is performed by asking the patient to name ten items in each of four categories: (1) fruits, (2) animals, (3) colors, and (4) towns (FACT is a helpful acronym). One point is given for each correct item and scoring is from 0 to 40.

In the original study, Isaacs and Kennie tested 189 individuals over age 65 who were also evaluated for dementia, intelligence, physical illness, affective disorder, and social class. They found that a score below 15 corresponded closely to a clinical diagnosis of dementia. No one scoring over 25 was found to be demented. Scores from 15 to 24 showed some association with dementia. Thus, a patient scoring less than 15, and possibly less than 25, should be thoroughly evaluated medically.

Mini-Mental State Exam: The Mini-Mental State Exam, like the Set Test, is a valid detector of organic disease in elderly patients (Folstein et al, 1975). The test requires five to ten minutes to administer and consists of 11 categories of questions with 30 responses. It is specifically a test of cognitive aspects of mental function and does not evaluate mood, logic, or abnormal mental experiences.

Folstein et al (1975) showed that this test is both reliable and valid. Patients with dementia had a mean score of 9.7; those with depression and secondary cognitive impairment (pseudodementia) had a mean score of 19; those with uncomplicated depression had a mean score of 25; and normals had a mean score of 27.6. They also showed that patients with pseudodementia raised their scores after treatment with antidepressants and/or electroconvulsive therapy.

Scores of 9 to 12 indicate a high likelihood of dementia and the need for a thorough medical evaluation, while scores of 25 and above predominate for normal subjects. The Mini-Mental State Exam is as follows (Keller and Manschreck, 1979):

1. Ask the patient to name the year, season, date, day, and month (5 points).
2. Ask the patient to name the state, county, town, hospital, and floor (5 points).
3. Ask the patient to repeat three unrelated objects that you name for him. Have him repeat these and continue to repeat them until he learns all three (3 points).
4. Have the patient subtract 7 from 100, stopping after five subtractions, or have him spell the word "world" backwards (5 points).
5. Ask the patient to repeat the three objects which he had previously been told (3 points).
6. Show the patient a wrist watch and ask him what it is. Repeat this for a pencil (2 points).
7. Ask the patient to repeat this phrase: "No ifs, ands, or buts!" (1 point).
8. Have the patient follow a three-point command such as, "Take a paper in your right hand, fold it in half, and put it on the floor!" (3 points).
9. On a blank piece of paper write the sentence, "Close your eyes!" Ask the patient to read it and do what it says (1 point).
10. Give the patient a blank piece of paper and ask him to write a sentence. It must be written spontaneously. Score correctly if it contains a subject and a verb and is sensible (1 point).
11. Ask the patient to copy a design that you have drawn for him

on a piece of paper. A good design is two intersecting pentagons with sides of about 1 inch each (1 point).

Total Possible = 30 points.

GUIDELINES FOR PRESCRIBING PSYCHOTROPIC DRUGS IN THE ELDERLY

A few general principles should be kept in mind when prescribing psychotropic drugs in the elderly:

1. *Careful history:* it is necessary to know what concomitant illnesses the patient has and it is crucial that the clinician know what medications have been taken. For instance, giving meperidine hydrochloride (Demerol) for pain relief to a patient experiencing a myocardial infarction who has been taking a monoamine oxidase inhibitor may be fatal. Many psychotropic agents produce anticholinergic effects which may add to an anticholinergic load from other agents such as antihistamines or cardiac antiarrhythmic agents.
2. *Diagnose prior to treatment:* This is imperative to avoid the inappropriate use of psychotropic medication. For example, if severe insomnia is secondary to a depression, benzodiazepines may worsen the overall clinical situation, while a sedating antidepressant will treat the underlying disorder. Treating uncomplicated anxiety with neuroleptics is inappropriate. A recent report of 42 patients with tardive dyskinesia seen in movement disorder clinics in various centers found that 19 had been inappropriately treated with neuroleptics (Burke et al, 1982). Of these, six patients had been treated for anxiety, six for depression, four for behavioral disturbances associated with mental retardation, and three for an acute psychotic episode precipitated by emotional stress.
3. *Evaluate potential for noncompliance:* Make the therapeutic regimen as simple as possible. Explain which medications are to be taken, the dosage, and the timing to both the patient and the family. Write down the dosing schedule. Choose the most appropriate dosage form; liquids may be more suitable for a patient with trouble swallowing. Encourage patients to destroy or return discontinued medication. In patients who are confused or demented, be sure that adequate supervision is present.
4. *Do not avoid the use of psychotropic agents just because of age:* these drugs can be used safely in the elderly, and older patients

deserve relief of symptoms of depression, psychosis, and severe anxiety. Avoiding the use of these agents, when they are required, contributes to suffering and may lead to death through suicide, malnutrition, and stress-related disorders.

5. *Use a low dose initially:* Because interindividual differences are so great in the elderly, the clinician should start with very low doses and titrate up gradually. Try to identify signs and symptoms which can be followed such as sleep disturbance, anorexia, hallucinations, or aggressive behavior. With some drugs, blood levels may be useful. Once a drug has reached steady-state levels, which takes about five half-lives, the plasma level may help the clinician determine whether enough drug is being given to achieve a therapeutic effect (Vestal, 1984).

6. *Know the pharmacology of the drug prescribed:* It is best to be familiar with the use of a few drugs in each class. The clinician needs to be aware of altered dosing schedules in the elderly and changes in half-life, elimination, and protein binding. Potential interactions with other drugs as well as toxicity and side effects must be kept in mind.

7. *Monitor drugs on a regular basis:* This is extremely important, especially when more than one physician may be prescribing medication or when neuroleptics are being used. It is not uncommon for medications to be continued for many months after the indication has resolved.

8. *Avoid polypharmacy:* not infrequently patients receive two or more drugs of the same type, or which have similar and additive side effects, perhaps prescribed by the same or different clinicians.

9. *Optimize the patient's environment:* Environmental manipulation may alleviate anxiety, loneliness, depression, and even psychosis. Optimize the patient's physical condition and encourage social activities and exercise whenever possible. Provide supportive individual and family psychotherapy when needed.

10. *Watch for drug side effects:* Most psychotropic agents have side effects which can be of major significance. Many of these may not be present when the drug is started and frequent monitoring is necessary.

REFERENCES

Bixler EO, Kales A, Soldatos CR, et al: Prevalence of sleep disorders in the Los Angeles metropolitan area. *Am J Psychiatry* 136:1257, 1979.
Burke RE, Fahn J, Janovic J, et al: Tardive dyskinesia and inappropriate use

of neuroleptic drugs. *Lancet* 1:1299, 1982.

Busse EW: The Duke Longitudinal Study. I:Senescence and senility, in Katzman R, et al (eds): *Alzheimer's Disease: Senile Dementia and Related Disorders.* New York, Raven Press, 1978.

Folstein MF, Folstein SE, McHugh PR: Mini-Mental State Exam: A practical method for grading the cognitive state of patients for the clinician. *J Psychiatry Res* 12:189–198, 1975.

Greenblatt DJ, Shader RI, Koch-Weser J: Psychotropic drug use in the Boston area: A report from the Boston Collaborative Drug Surveillance Program. *Arch Gen Psychiatry* 32:518–523, 1975.

Guttmann D: A study of drug-taking behavior of older Americans, in Beber CR, Lamy PP (eds): *Medication Management and Education in the Elderly.* Amsterdam, Excerpta Medica, 1978.

Isaacs B, Kennie AT: The Set Test as an aid to the detection of dementia in old people. *Br J Psychiatry* 123:467–470, 1973.

Jenike MA: Treatable dementias. *Topics in Geriatrics* 1(1):1–2, 1982.

Keller MB, Manschreck TC: The biologic mental status examination, in Lazare A (ed): *Outpatient Psychiatry.* Baltimore, Williams & Wilkins Co, 1979, pp 203–214.

19% of Americans have mental illness NIMH finds. *Psychiatric News* Nov 2, 1984, p.1.

Parry HJ, Balter MB, Mellinger GD, et al: National patterns of psychotherapeutic drug use. *Arch Gen Psychiatry* 28:769–776, 1973.

Pfeiffer E: The psychosocial evaluation of the elderly patient, in Busse EW, Blazer DG (eds): *Handbook of Geriatric Psychiatry.* New York, Van Nostrand Reinhold Co, 1980, pp 275–284.

Salzman C: *Clinical Geriatric Psychopharmacology.* New York, McGraw-Hill Book Co, 1984.

Vestal RE (ed): *Drug Treatment in the Elderly.* Boston, ADIS Health Science Press, 1984.

Wilson LA, Lawson IR, Braws W: Multiple disorders in the elderly. A clinical and statistical study. *Lancet* 2:841–847, 1962.

"Aging is when the gleam in your eyes is from the sun hitting your bifocals."

CHAPTER **2**

Altered Drug Metabolism

In order to use psychopharmacologic agents wisely in the elderly patient, certain physiologic concomitants of aging should be kept in mind. These include changes in drug absorption, distribution, protein binding, hepatic metabolism, and renal excretion (Table 2-1). Changes in receptor sensitivity and brain neurotransmitters are also recently being reported (Jenike, 1982a; Vestal, 1984; Greenblatt et al, 1982; Salzman, 1984).

AGE-RELATED CHANGES

Absorption

Overall, changes in absorption are the least important physiologic alterations accompanying aging. In general, gastric pH is higher and intestinal blood flow is reduced. Also, gastric emptying is delayed, gastrointestinal (GI) motility is decreased, and the number of absorbing

Table 2-1
Altered Metabolism with Aging

Absorption
Distribution
Protein binding
Hepatic metabolism
Renal excretion
Receptor sensitivity
Brain enzyme systems
    Decreased acetylcholine and dopamine
    Increased monoamine oxidase

cells is lower in the elderly. Decreased active transport in the elderly is well documented, but since most psychotropic agents are passively diffused, this has little or no effect. Clearly, more research is needed in this area, but the available data suggest that age alone produces few changes on the gut which are of clinical significance in terms of drug metaboism (Plein and Plein, 1981; Schumacher, 1980).

Distribution

Distribution changes are, on the other hand, clinically very important in the elderly. On the average, elderly patients tend to be smaller than younger patients and standard drug doses might be expected to result in higher blood and tissue levels (Greenblatt et al, 1982).

As we age, total body water decreases, lean body mass is reduced, and body fat increases (Bruce et al, 1980; Novak, 1972; Forbes and Reina, 1970). From age 20 to 60 years, body water levels may decrease from 25% to 18%. Drugs such as ethanol which are distributed in body water will have higher levels in an elderly person because of an apparent decrease in the size of their reservoir (Vestal et al, 1977). In the same period, the proportion of total body fat may increase from 10% to 50% (Greenblatt et al, 1982). This increases the volume of distribution of lipid-soluble drugs, such as desmethyldiazepam, a metabolite of diazepam (Valium), and contributes to greatly prolonged drug half-life (Greenblatt et al, 1980; Allen et al, 1980; Greenblatt et al, 1981). From Figure 2-1, it can be seen that drug half-life is raised by an elevation of the volume of distribution or by a decrease in creatinine clearance (Greenblatt et al, 1982). As a consequence of changes in volume of distribution and clearance, the half-life of diazepam metabolites is prolonged from an average of 20 hours at age 20 to 90 hours at age 80 (Rosenbaum, 1979).

$$T\frac{1}{2} = \frac{Vd \times K}{Ccl}$$

where T½ = half-life
Vd = volume of distribution
K = constant
Ccl = creatinine clearance

Figure 2-1 Relation of drug half-life to volume of distribution and renal clearance.

Serum albumin levels are reduced by 15% to 25% in the elderly (Schumacher, 1980; Bender et al, 1975; Hayes et al, 1975). Since many psychotropic drugs bind to albumin, this is clinically important. Free drug concentration is an important determinant of drug distribution, elimination, and action. The less albumin available for drug binding, the more free drug is available to body tissues where sites of action may be located. Increased free drug may make the elderly patient more susceptible to adverse effects or more vulnerable to the effects of multiple drug therapy on drug binding. Some experts feel that this age difference itself does not change clinical drug effects, as the free drug concentration at steady state is a function of dose and clearance, not the unbound fraction itself (Greenblatt et al, 1982).

Hepatic Metabolism

Psychotropic drugs are primarily removed from the circulation by the liver, which produces active and inactive metabolites, and by the kidney which excretes some unchanged drugs as well as hepatic metabolites.

In persons over 65, hepatic blood flow is decreased by 40% compared to a person aged 25 years (Bender, 1965; Geokas and Haverback, 1969). This is at least partially the result of an age-associated decline in cardiac output. In addition, liver size in relation to body mass decreases with age (Vestal, 1984).

Antipyrine is useful for studying hepatic metabolism as it is minimally protein-bound and is largely metabolized by the liver (Vestal, 1984). One large study of antipyrine metabolism revealed an interindividual variation of sixfold in similarly aged subjects (Vestal et al, 1975). Only 3% of the variance in liver metabolic clearance could be explained by age alone. These data confirm the frequent clinical impression that no consistent generalizations hold true in reference to hepatic metabolism in the elderly (Jenike, 1982a; 1983). Frequently we see 80-year-old patients who require doses comparable to those given to 25-year-old patients. For example, some elderly patients reach therapeutic levels of desipramine hydrochloride (Norpramin, Pertofrane) on a daily dose of 25 mg while others may require 200 mg.

The metabolism of most psychotropic drugs is primarily by the hepatic microsomal enzymes (Veith, 1984). Tobacco smoking may cause less induction of the microsomal enzymes in the elderly than in younger patients (Vestal and Wood, 1980). Long-term alcohol use can induce liver microsomal activity and increase the rate of psychotropic drug metabolism after alcohol is out of the system. While alcohol is still in the blood, microsomal enzymes are inhibited (Vestal et al, 1977; Sellers and Holloway, 1978; Sellers et al, 1980; Sandor et al, 1981).

Renal Excretion

In contrast to the variable and unpredictable changes in hepatic metabolism, renal concomitants of aging are well studied, easily measured, and consistent. The glomerular filtration rate (GFR) decreases by approximately 50% by age 70 (Papper, 1978). Over the period from 20 to 80 years of age, there is a 20% decrease in kidney size and a 30% loss in the number of functional glomeruli (Davies and Shock, 1950; Rowe, 1978). The creatinine clearance of the healthy kidneys declines by 0.5 to 1.0 mL/min/1.73 m²/yr. Renal plasma flow also declines during these years by 1.5% to 2.0%/yr (Bender, 1965; Schumacher, 1980). If kidney damage or disease are superimposed on these normal changes, it will enhance the age-related reduced clearance. For drugs whose clearance is partly or entirely by renal excretion of the intact drug, clearance will predictably decline approximately in proportion to the reduced GFR.

Serum creatinine alone is often a poor guide to the evaluation of renal status in the elderly since it may be normal in the face of greatly reduced renal function. Lean body mass decreases with age and produces a concomitant lowering of the daily creatinine production. Since the serum creatinine concentration depends on creatinine production as well as renal creatinine clearance, a decline in renal function in an elderly patient may not yield an elevated creatinine concentration. Creatinine clearance based on 24-hour urinary excretion, as well as on serum creatinine concentration, is a far more accurate indicator of kidney function (Greenblatt et al, 1982). Figure 2-2 gives an often used formula to estimate true creatinine clearance in relation to age in men. For women, multiply the computed creatinine clearance by 0.85 (Jenike, 1982b).

Changes in renal excretion are known to be important for digoxin, procainamide, penicillins, and aminoglycosides (Jenike, 1982b; Greenblatt et al, 1982). It is less well known, however, that long-acting benzodiazepine metabolism is profoundly altered by age-related changes in renal clearance. For example, as mentioned earlier, the half-lives of diazepam metabolites are increased from an average of 20 hours at age 20 to 90 hours at age 80, largely due to changes in renal excretion. Lithium carbonate (Eskalith and others), a drug with a very limited range of tolerable plasma levels, undergoes over a 30% reduction in

$$Ccl = \frac{(140 - age) \times body\ weight\ (kg)}{72 \times serum\ creatinine}$$

(for women, multiply computed Ccl by 0.85)

Figure 2-2 Computing creatinine clearance (Ccl).

renal clearance when comparing patients age 25 to those age 75 (Lehman and Merten, 1974); Roughlerten, 1974). Roughly a one-third reduction in dosage is needed to maintain comparable blood levels in the elderly (Hewick and Newbury, 1976).

RECEPTOR SENSITIVITY
AND NEUROTRANSMITTERS

Much research is being directed to understanding age-related changes in receptors and brain neurotransmitters (Salzman, 1984). In theory, a reduced sensitivity to pharmacologic response could be postulated as a result of a decreased number of receptors, decreased availability of enzymes to mediate the effect of the drug, and increased resistance to drug diffusion through tissues. Studies with isoproterenol hydrochloride (Isuprel) and propranolol hydrochloride (Inderal) indicate that the elderly are indeed more resistant to the effects of these two compounds (London et al, 1976; Vestal et al, 1979). The dose of isoproterenol needed to increase the heart rate by 25 beats per minute is four to six times higher in old persons as compared to young (Vestal et al, 1979). On the other hand, many drugs demonstrate a heightened response with age. Common examples include the effects of sedatives (Reidenberg et al, 1978; Giles et al, 1978), narcotics (Bellville et al, 1971; Kaiko, 1980), and anticoagulants (Husted and Andreasen, 1977; Shepherd et al, 1977; Hotraphinyo et al, 1978).

There are reports of decreased CNS dopamine and acetylcholine which may make the elderly more sensitive to drug side effects (Robinson et al, 1972; Horita, 1978). Alzheimer's victims have striking loss of cholinergic cells in the basal forebrain, and the enzyme choline acetyltransferase, responsible for the production of acetylcholine, is drastically reduced in their brains (Davies, 1979; Jenike, 1984a). Thus, any drug with anticholinergic effects will further impair an already damaged system.

As we age, most neurotransmitters and enzyme levels seem to decrease (Goodnick and Gershon, 1984). Recently, however, it has been demonstrated that there is a marked increase in monoamine oxidase (MAO) levels with age in human plasma, platelets, and brain (Gottfries et al, 1983). Norepinephrine concentrations correlate negatively and 5-hydroxyindoleacetic acid concentrations correlate positively with brainstem MAO activity (Jenike, 1985). This suggests that MAO plays a major role in regulating intracellular biogenic amines. There is a linear decrease of norepinephrine levels with age and this is consistent with the hypothesis that these age-related decrements in norepinephrine levels are a consequence of the also age-related increase in MAO activity (Jenike, 1985). If biogenic amines are indeed lowered by increased MAO in elderly patients, this could lead to states of low central norepinephrine and/or serotonin which could make the elderly particularly vulnerable to depression. This age-related increase in MAO activity has been shown to be even more pronounced in demented patients and it has been suggested that MAO inhibitors (MAOI) may be particularly useful in treating depressed Alzheimer's patients (Jenike, 1984; 1985) (see chapter 4).

SUMMARY

With aging, there are major changes in the body which affect the manner in which psychopharmacologic agents are metabolized. Changes in absorption are of little importance. Changes in hepatic metabolism are variable with aging and interindividual differences far outweigh age-related alterations. On the other hand, alterations in drug distribution, renal function, and brain enzyme systems and neurotransmitters are consistent and of major consequence. In contrast to most brain enzyme systems, monoamine oxidase is increased and this may have important consequences, such as an increased tendency for the elderly, particularly those who are demented, to suffer from clinical depression.

REFERENCES

Allen MD, Greenblatt DJ, Harmatz JS, et al: Desmethyldiazepam kinetics in the elderly after oral prazepam. *Clin Pharmacol Ther* 28:196–202, 1980.

Bellville JW, Forrest WH, Miller E, et al: Influence of age on pain relief from analgesics: A study of postoperative patients. *JAMA* 217:1835–1841, 1971.

Bender AD: The effect of increasing age on the distribution of peripheral blood flow in man. *J Am Geriatr Soc* 13:192–198, 1965.

Bender AD, Post A, Meier JP, et al: Plasma protein binding of drugs as a function of age in adult human subjects. *J Pharm Sci* 64:1711–1713, 1975.

Bruce A, Anderson M, Arvidsson B, et al: Body composition. Prediction of normal body potassium, body water and body fat in adults on the basis of body height, body weight and age. *Scand J Clin Lab Invest* 40:461–473, 1980.

Davies DF, Shock N: Age changes in glomerular filtration rate, effective renal plasma flow, and the tubular excretory capacity in adult males. *J Clin Invest* 29:496, 1950.

Davies P: Neurotransmitter-related symptoms in SDAT. *Brain Res* 171:319, 1979.

Forbes GB, Reina JC: Adult lean body mass declines with age: Some longitudinal observations. *Metabolism* 19:653–663, 1970.

Geokas MC, Haverback BJ: The aging gastrointestinal tract. *Am J Surg* 117:881–892, 1969.

Giles HG, MacLeod SM, Wright JR, et al: Influence of age and previous use on diazepam dosage required for endoscopy. *Can Med Assoc J* 118:513–514, 1978.

Goodnick P, Gershon S: Chemotherapy of cognitive disorders in geriatric subjects. *J Clin Psychiatry* 45:196–209, 1984.

Gottfries CG, Adolfsson R, Aquilonius SM, et al: Biochemical changes in dementia disorders of Alzheimer's type (AD/SDAT). *Neurobiol Aging* 4:261–271, 1983.

Greenblatt DJ, Allen MD, Harmatz JS, et al: Diazepam disposition determinants. *Clin Pharmacol Ther* 27:301–312, 1980.

Greenblatt DJ, Divoll M, Puri SK, et al: Clobazam kinetics in the elderly. *Br J Clin Pharmacol* 12:631–636, 1981.

Greenblatt DJ, Sellers EM, Shader RI: Drug disposition in old age. *N Engl J Med* 306:1081–1088, 1982.

Hayes MJ, Langman MJS, Short AH: Changes in drug metabolism with increasing age: phenytoin clearance and protein binding. *Br J Clin Pharmacol* 2:73-79, 1975.

Hewick DS, Newbury PA: Age: Its influence on lithium dosage and plasma levels. *Br J Clin Pharmacol* 3:354, 1976.

Horita A: Neuropharmacology and aging, in Roberts J, Adelman RC, Cristatalo VJ (eds): *Pharmacological Intervention in the Aging Process*. New York, Plenum Press, 1978.

Hotraphinyo K, Triggs EJ, Maybloom B, et al: Warfarin sodium: Steady-state plasma levels and patient age. *Clin Exp Pharmacol Physiol* 5:143–149, 1978.

Husted S, Andreasen F: The influence of age on the response to anticoagulants. *Br J Clin Pharmacol* 4:559–565, 1977.

Jenike MA: Using sedative drugs in the elderly. *Drug Therapy* 12:186–190, 1982a.

Jenike MA: Using digoxin in the elderly. *Topics in Geriatrics* 1:21–23, 1982b.

Jenike MA: Treatment of anxiety in elderly patients. *Geriatrics* 38:115–120, 1983.

Jenike MA: Monoamine oxidase inhibitors in elderly depressed patients. *J Am Ger Soc* 32:571-575, 1984.

Jenike MA: MAO inhibitors as treatment for depressed patients with primary degenerative dementia (Alzheimer's disease). *Am J Psychiatry* (in press).

Kaiko RF: Age and morphine analgesia in cancer patients with postoperative pain. *Clin Pharmacol Ther* 28:823–827, 1980.

Lehman K, Merten X: Die Elimination von Lithium in Abhängigkeit vom Lebensalter bei Gesunden und Niereninsuffizienten. *Int J Clin Pharmacol Ther Toxicol* 10:292–298, 1974.

London GM, Safar ME, Weiss YA, et al: Isoproterenol sensitivity and total body clearance of propranolol in hypertensive patients. *J Clin Pharmacol* 16:174–179, 1976.

Novak LP: Aging, total body potassium, fat-free mass, and cell mass in males and females between ages 18 and 35 years. *J Gerontol* 27:438–443, 1972.

Papper S: *Clinical Nephrology*. Boston, Little Brown & Company, 1978.

Plein JB, Plein EM: Aging and drug therapy, in Eisdorfer C (ed): *Annual Review of Gerontology and Geriatrics*. New York, Springer-Verlag, vol 2, p 211, 1981.

Reidenberg MM, Levy M, Warner H, et al: Relationship between diazepam dose, plasma level, age, and central nervous system depression. *Clin Pharmacol Ther* 23:371–374, 1978.

Robinson DS, Davis JM, Nies A, et al: Aging, monoamines and MAO levels. *Lancet* 1:290–291, 1972.

Rosenbaum JF: Anxiety, in Lazare A (ed): *Outpatient Psychiatry*. Baltimore, Williams & Wilkins Co, 1979, pp 252–256.

Rowe JW: The influence of age on renal function. *Res Staff Phys* 24:49–55, 1978.

Salzman C: Neurotransmission in the aging central nervous system, in Salzman C (ed): *Clinical Geriatric Psychopharmacology*. New York, McGraw-Hill Book Co, 1984, pp 18–31.

Sandor P, Sellers EM, Dumbrell M, et al: Effect of short- and long-term alcohol use on phenytoin kinetics in chronic alcoholics. *Clin Pharmacol Ther* 30:390–397, 1981.

Schumacher GE: Using pharmacokinetics in drug therapy: VII: Pharmacokinetic factors influencing drug therapy in the aged. *Am J Hosp Pharm* 37:559–562, 1980.

Sellers EM, Giles HG, Greenblatt DJ, et al: Differential effects on benzodiazepine disposition by disulfiram and ethanol. *Arzneimittelforsch* 30:882–886, 1980.

Sellers EM, Holloway MR: Drug kinetics and alcohol ingestion. *Clin Pharmacokinet* 3:440–452, 1978.

Shepherd AMM, Hewick DS, Moreland TA, et al: Age as a determinant of sensitivity to warfarin. *Br J Clin Pharmacol* 4:315–320, 1977.

Veith RC: Treatment of psychiatric disorders, in Vestal RE (ed): *Drug Treatment in the Elderly*. Boston, ADIS Health Science Press, 1984, pp 317–337.

Vestal RE: Geriatric clinical pharmacology: An overview, in Vestal RE (ed): *Drug Treatment in the Elderly*. Boston, ADIS Health Science Press, 1984, pp 12–28.

Vestal RE, McGuire EA, Tobin JD, et al: Aging and ethanol metabolism. *Clin Pharmacol Ther* 21:343–354, 1977.

Vestal RE, Norris AH, Tobin JD, et al: Antipyrine metabolism in man: Influence of age, alcohol, caffeine, and smoking. *Clin Pharmacol Ther* 18:425–434, 1975.

Vestal RE, Wood AJJ, Shand DG: Reduced β-adrenoreceptor sensitivity in the elderly. *Clin Pharmacol Ther* 26:181–186, 1979.

Vestal RE, Wood AJJ: Influence of age and smoking on drug kinetics in man: Studies using model compounds. *Clin Pharmacokinetics* 5:309–318, 1980.

"Aging is when you sink your teeth into a steak and they stay there."

CHAPTER 3

Psychosis, Rage, and Violence

Elderly patients who are psychotic, violent, or exhibit inappropriately aggressive behavior are particularly disruptive and present a therapeutic challenge to the clinician. The medications used to control such symptoms are, on the one hand, very effective, but on the other, are likely to produce side effects of a serious nature. Patients who require major tranquilizers or neuroleptics usually fall into a few general categories. The majority of such patients suffer from moderate to severe dementia while a smaller percentage may have a lifelong psychotic process. Many schizophrenics live into old age and, with the present thrust towards deinstitutionalization, they are finding their way into nursing homes or are living in the community. Disturbances of behavior and thinking are also present in the delirious or acutely confused patient as well as in some elderly patients whose affective illnesses have reached psychotic proportions.

TREATMENT

Neuroleptics

In the early 1950s, chlorpromazine (Thorazine) was introduced into the United States for clinical use. This was a major breakthrough because prior to the introduction of chlorpromazine, psychotic symptoms were managed by sedation only. The neuroleptics were found to be capable of controlling many of the clinical signs and symptoms of psychosis such as aggressive and disordered behavior, hallucinations, delusions, paranoia, and disordered thinking.

All of the currently available neuroleptics have the ability to block dopamine and considerable clinical and laboratory evidence suggests that their clinical potency parallels their dopamine blocking power

Table 3-1
Equivalent Doses of Neuroleptics

| Generic Name | Trade Name | Side Effects | | | Approximate Equivalent Dose (mg) |
		Sedative	Anti-Cholinergic	Extra-Pyramidal	
Low Potency					
Chlorpromazine	Thorazine	High	High	Low	100
Thioridazine	Mellaril	High	High	Low	95
Intermediate Potency					
Perphenazine	Trilafon	Moderate	Moderate	Moderate	10
Loxapine Succinate	Loxitane	Moderate	Moderate	Moderate	15
Molindone HCl	Moban	Moderate	Moderate	Moderate	10
High Potency					
Haloperidol	Haldol	Low	Low	High	2
Thiothixene	Navane	Low	Low	High	5
Fluphenazine HCl	Prolixin	Low	Low	High	2
Trifluoperazine HCl	Stelazine	Moderate	Low	Moderate	5

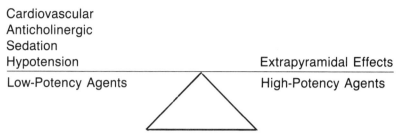

Cardiovascular
Anticholinergic
Sedation
Hypotension   Extrapyramidal Effects
Low-Potency Agents   High-Potency Agents

Figure 3-1   Balancing neuroleptic side effects.

(Snyder et al, 1974; Bernstein, 1978). Their antipsychotic effects are independent of their sedative potential.

Choosing a neuroleptic   Neuroleptic agents have a wide range of potencies (Table 3-1) and can be roughly separated into three groups based on antipsychotic potency. As can be seen from Table 3-1, 2 mg of haloperidol (Haldol) is roughly equivalent to 100 mg of chlorpromazine. As with antidepressants, the various neuroleptics are generally considered to be equally effective and the choice of medication should be based on predicted type of side effects.

Low-potency agents, such as chlorpromazine and thioridazine (Mellaril), produce significant sedation, orthostatic hypotension, and anticholinergic effects (Jenike, 1982a). On the other hand, high-potency drugs such as haloperidol and fluphenazine hydrochloride (Prolixin) are much more likely to cause extrapyramidal side effects such as dystonia, akathisia, and parkinsonism (Figure 3-1). Haloperidol produces negligible cardiovascular side effects even when used intravenously (Sos and Cassem, 1980).

Neuroleptics are also potent α-adrenergic blocking agents and produce peripheral vasodilatation and hypotension. Chlorpromazine and thioridazine (low-potency agents) are most likely to cause hypotension. This effect is so profound that chlorpromazine is even used to treat hypertensive crises induced by MAO inhibitor–tyramine interactions (see chapter 4). Haloperidol has the least α-blocking ability of the currently available antipsychotic drugs and is the preferred agent in the very elderly or frail patient. Since falls are devastating in the very elderly, high-potency agents such as haloperidol, thiothixene (Navane), and fluphenazine are safer because they are less likely to induce hypotensive episodes (Figure 3-1).

Unfortunately, when using the high-potency agents, which produce fewer cardiovascular effects, the physician is more likely to induce extrapyramidal side effects. These can occasionally be very disabling especially in patients with pre-existing extrapyramidal illness such as Parkinson's disease. In such cases, very low doses of chlorpromazine or thioridazine (ie, 10 mg twice daily initially) may produce the desired effect without further compromising motor status.

If the high-potency agents are used cautiously in low dosage (ie, haloperidol 0.5 mg or thiothixene 1.0 mg twice daily initially), the possibility of unwanted extrapyramidal effects can be minimized. Extrapyramidal reactions are uncommon at very low dosages but will commonly occur if doses must be increased to control symptoms. Extrapyramidal reactions, even if they do occur, are less likely to produce serious clinical problems than excessive drowsiness, cardiac effects, or severe hypotension in a geriatric patient.

Side effects Neuroleptics have a number of side effects. These will be reviewed briefly. The elderly commonly develop sedation, orthostatic hypotension, anticholinergic signs and symptoms, and extrapyramidal effects. Some of the age-related metabolic changes have been reviewed in chapter 2.

1. *Anticholinergic side effects:* Anticholinergic side effects, toxicity, diagnosis, and treatment are reviewed in chapter 8. The peripheral anticholinergic effects are generally less pronounced than those induced by the tricyclic antidepressants. In in vitro studies the *least* anticholinergic tricyclic, desipramine, is about equipotent to the *most* anticholinergic neuroleptic, thioridazine (see Table 8-1).

We now know that the cholinergic system is intimately involved in memory (Drachman and Leavitt, 1974) and that in Alzheimer's disease there is a loss of cholinergic neurons and decrements in the enzyme choline acetyltransferase which is responsible for the production of central acetylcholine (Davies, 1979). The anticholinergic side effects of neuroleptic drugs in the presence of age-related decreases in cholinergic functioning can lead to serious problems in the elderly patient. When anticholinergic agents are given to treat neuroleptic-induced extrapyramidal problems, the likelihood of side effects increases. It is important that the clinician be aware of all medications that his/her elderly patient is taking, as anticholinergic effects are additive (see chapter 8).

2. *Ophthalmologic side effects:* The most serious eye problem related to neuroleptic usage is the irreversible degenerative pigmentary retinopathy caused by thioridazine in doses in excess of 800 mg/day (Baldessarini, 1977). In addition, reversible deposits of drug substances and pigment in the lens and cornea have been associated with long-term neuroleptic usage.

3. *Photosensitivity:* Patients taking neuroleptics are sometimes un-

usually sensitive to the sun. Maculopapular rashes occur on occasion and sometimes a blue-gray discoloration of the skin results, usually with prolonged high doses of chlorpromazine (Baldessarini, 1977). Photosensitivity is managed by decreased solar exposure and by sun screens.

4. *Temperature regulation dysfunction:* Neuroleptics may upset hypothalamic thermoregulatory mechanisms and make the elderly patient more vulnerable to either excessive heat or cold. This side effect is particularly dangerous in the south in the summer and in the north in the winter — where many elderly patients are surviving on low incomes and have to choose between food and heat or air conditioning.

5. *Hematologic side effects:* Hematologic complications of neuroleptic use are very rare. Frank agranulocytosis occurs infrequently (incidence less than 0.01%) and has a peak incidence within the first two months of treatment (Baldessarini, 1977). Agranulocytosis is most common in elderly females and is almost always associated with the use of low-potency agents. It is virtually unknown with haloperidol (Baldessarini, 1977). Agranulocytosis is a life-threatening medical emergency which can rarely be predicted from occasional white blood cell counts and must be suspected whenever fever, sore throat, or malaise occur early in the course of neuroleptic treatment. When diagnosed, the drug must be immediately discontinued and the patient hospitalized for reverse isolation. If a life-threatening infection does not supervene, agranulocytosis is usually reversible within a few weeks (Gelenberg, 1978).

6. *Jaundice:* Neuroleptic-induced jaundice is almost always an allergic cholestatic type, is usually transient, and is usually caused by phenothiazines such as chlorpromazine. As modern technology has allowed for greater drug purity, this complication is exceedingly rare. Older patients with a history of obstructive jaundice or liver disease should not be treated with this class of drug (Spira et al, 1984).

7. *Weight gain:* Weight gain is sometimes seen in association with neuroleptic use. This is particularly troublesome to some patients, particularly those who are already overweight. It is reported that molindone hydrochloride (Lidone, Moban) is less likely than other neuroleptics to induce an increase in body weight (Gelenberg, 1978).

8. *Cardiovascular effects:* Cardiac effects are rarely a problem with high-potency antipsychotic agents. Orthostatic hypotension can be induced by the less potent phenothiazines. Thioridazine is known to have the strongest effects of any of the antipsychotic drugs on cardiac conduction and repolarization (Gelenberg, 1978). Neuroleptic drugs, particularly thioridazine, can produce nonspecific T-wave changes on the ECG which are of no clinical significance. Because of its effect on

cardiac conduction, thioridazine should probably not be used in the presence of conduction defects or other cardiac disease, or in conjunction with drugs with similar cardiac actions such as the tricyclic antidepressants, quinidine, or procainamide (Gelenberg, 1978).

9. *Seizures:* Neuroleptics, especially low-potency agents, may increase the incidence of seizures in epileptic patients (Baldessarini, 1977) or in patients with pre-existing CNS pathology (Spira et al, 1984). In the elderly, obtaining a careful history of previous seizures is mandatory and dosage increases in susceptible patients should be very slow. High-potency agents such as haloperidol may have less tendency to induce seizures (Baldessarini, 1977).

10. *Sedation:* Drowsiness is often seen early in therapy and is much more prominent with the low-potency agents. Tolerance to sedation does seem to develop over a few weeks. Early in therapy, sedation can be advantageous for daytime calming or to promote sleep.

11. *Syndrome of inappropriate secretion of antidiuretic hormone (SIADH):* Both high- and low-potency neuroleptics have been associated with SIADH (Matuk and Kalyanaraman, 1977; Rivera, 1975; Rao et al, 1975; Husband et al, 1981; Miller and Moses, 1976). Whenever patients taking neuroleptics show deterioration of their behavior, with irritability, personality changes, or progressive alteration of sensorium, SIADH must be considered in the differential diagnosis. This condition is not rare and can be easily diagnosed with simple tests of serum and urine osmolality. Bartter has outlined five criteria for the diagnosis of this syndrome: (*a*) hyponatremia and hypo-osmolality of extracellular fluids, (*b*) persistence of sodium in the urine despite hyponatremia, (*c*) absence of signs of dehydration, (*d*) normal renal function, and (*e*) normal adrenal function. Simple water intoxication arising from a large intake of water may occur in psychotics (Raskind, 1974), but if antidiuretic hormone (ADH) secretion is appropriately suppressed, the urinary osmolality will be at the minimal possible value (Bartter, 1973).

12. *Extrapyramidal reactions:* A number of extrapyramidal reactions can occur with the use of neuroleptics. These are presumably due to the dopamine blocking power of these agents on the basal ganglia and the rest of the extrapyramidal motor system. For example, the frequently occurring drug-induced parkinsonian syndrome may reflect the ability of the antipsychotic agents to block the action of dopamine as a synaptic neurotransmitter in the caudate nucleus, much as spontaneously occurring parkinsonism reflects the degeneration of the dopamine-mediated nigrostriatal pathway from midbrain to the caudate nucleus (Baldessarini, 1977). Clinicians must be aware of several discrete extrapyramidal syndromes which can be associated with the use of neu-

roleptic agents. They include acute dystonias, parkinsonism and akathisia, tardive dyskinesia, withdrawal dyskinesias, and catatonic reaction.

a. *Dystonias:* The acute dystonias are exceedingly uncommon in the elderly but occur frequently in the young — particularly in males. These occur within the first few days of treatment and involve distressing tonic contractions of the muscles of the neck, mouth, and tongue. Opisthotonus and oculogyric crises also sometimes occur. These reactions are frequently misdiagnosed as hysterical or as a psychotic symptom. Treatment is almost always rapidly effective and involves parenteral injection of an anticholinergic agent. Diphenhydramine hydrochloride (Benadryl) 25 mg intramuscularly (IM) or intravenously (IV) or benztropine mesylate (Cogentin) 1 to 2 mg IV will result in rapid relief.

b. *Parkinsonism:* Drug-induced parkinsonism is commonly seen in the elderly and cannot be distinguished clinically from idiopathic Parkinson's disease. A history of neuroleptic intake must be obtained in order to make the diagnosis. The typical patient with drug-induced parkinsonism will exhibit slowed movements (bradykinesia) and muscular rigidity, stooped posture, shuffling gait, inexpressive masklike face, tremor, and drooling. This syndrome usually occurs after the first week to two months after neuroleptic treatment is begun. Tolerance probably develops to this symptom complex and the symptoms may fade over two to three months allowing the reduction and eventual discontinuing of antiparkinsonian agents. Besides the anticholinergic agents such as benztropine, diphenhydramine, and trihexyphenidyl hydrochloride (Artane), amantadine hydrochloride (Symmetrel) in doses of 100 to 300 mg daily is frequently effective in reversing parkinsonian side effects. Because of the dangers inherent in giving anticholinergic agents to the elderly (see chapter 8), amantadine is frequently used as the drug of first choice in treating such reactions in the elderly.

c. *Akathisia:* Another neuroleptic-induced extrapyramidal side effect is akathisia. It involves motor restlessness, pacing, inability to sit still, and a pressure to move about. This is associated with a subjective sensation of discomfort which is often described as anxiety. Sleep is usually disturbed because the individual is unable to find a comfortable motionless position. Sometimes this restlessness is misinterpretated as an increase in psychotic symptomatology and is inappropriately treated with an increase in neuroleptic dosage. It has been reported that the syndrome of neuroleptic-induced akathisia can even cause a worsening of the psychotic syndrome for which the neuroleptic treatment was initially being used (Van Putten et al, 1974; Van Putten, 1975).

One of the most effective treatments for akathisia has been lowering the dose of the offending neuroleptic. Other treatments that have been reportedly successful include anticholinergic agents (Van Putten et al, 1974), benzdiazepines (Ekbom, 1965), and amantadine (DiMascio et al, 1976). These agents are, however, frequently ineffective. A recent report by Lipinski and colleagues (1984) described an open trial of propranolol in 14 patients with neuroleptic-induced akathisia. Their decision to try propranolol for this disorder was based on an earlier report in which restless leg syndrome (an idiopathic disorder resembling akathisia) was reported to respond to treatment with propranolol (Ekbom, 1944; Strang, 1967). Lipinski et al found that all 14 patients demonstrated substantial improvement of their akathisia; nine obtained complete relief. The maximum therapeutic result was often obtained within 24 hours of starting propranolol. Doses were quite low and ranged from 30 to 80 mg/day. It is worthy of note that patients experienced no improvement in symptoms of either parkinsonism or tardive dyskinesia. On the basis of this preliminary uncontrolled trial, it does appear that propranolol may be of considerable benefit in the treatment of neuroleptic-induced akathisia. It seems very unlikely that improvement was due to a placebo effect, because ten of the 14 patients previously received benztropine without result.

d. *Catatonia:* Rarely, elderly patients will become unresponsive and catatonic after very low doses of neuroleptic. This may respond rapidly to IV doses of diphenhydramine or benztropine. After resolution of the acute episode, anticholinergic agents or amantadine may be helpful in preventing recurrence.

e. *Withdrawal dyskinesia:* Another infrequent extrapyramidal reaction is the induction of a withdrawal dyskinesia when neuroleptics are tapered rapidly or discontinued. This usually occurs after discontinuation of high doses of neuroleptic. Abrupt withdrawal of large neuroleptic doses is very frequently complicated by acute choreoathetotic reactions, similar in appearance to tardive dyskinesia, but usually lasting for only a few days. Withdrawal dyskinesias require no treatment and probably represent a transient rebound increase in the activity of previously inhibited dopaminergic neurons in the basal ganglia (Baldessarini, 1977).

f. *Tardive dyskinesia:* Tardive dyskinesia is manifested by a wide variety of movements, including lip smacking, sucking, jaw movements, flycatcher's tongue, writhing tongue movements, chorea, athetosis, dystonia, tics, and facial grimacing (Jenike, 1983a). In severe cases, speech, eating, walking, and even breathing can be seriously impaired. The disorder usually has a gradual onset after long-term, high-dose antipsychotic drug administration, but on rare occasions it can occur in patients who have had short-term or low-dose administration (Baldessarini, 1977). It is becoming increasingly clear that elderly patients are at very high risk of developing tardive dyskinesia after neuroleptic use. Many risk factors for tardive dyskinesia have been studied, including cumulative drug exposure, maximum neuroleptic dose, length of drug exposure, age, sex, drug type, polypharmacy, presence of organic mental disorder, prior use of anticholinergic antiparkinsonian drugs, presence or absence of drug-free intervals, and diagnosis of the patient. Recently, Kane and Smith (1982) reviewed 56 studies comprising almost 35,000 patients who were treated with neuroleptics; they found a mean prevalence of tardive dyskinesia uncorrected for spontaneous dyskinesias of 20%. They also reviewed 19 studies involving 11,000 patients who were never treated with neuroleptics and found a 5% incidence of spontaneous dyskinesias. These figures suggest that abnormal involuntary movements may have developed in some treated persons for reasons other than neuroleptic exposure. A best estimate of true drug-induced tardive dyskinesia is about 15% (20% prevalence in neuroleptic treated patients minus 5% spontaneous rate). Exposure to neuroleptics almost certainly plays a highly significant role in the production of abnormal involuntary movements. Of all the risk factor previously mentioned, only age and female sex have a relatively consistent effect in increasing the prevalence of tardive dyskinesia.

Smith and Baldessarini (1980) also found that advancing age correlated not only with increased prevalence but also with the severity of tardive dyskinesia. In addition, they observed diminishing rates of spontaneous remission of tardive dyskinesia after neuroleptics were discontinued in elderly patients. The correlation between age and the degree of remission after discontinuance of neuroleptics was highly significant. After cessation of neuroleptic therapy, the rate of improvement was 83% for patients younger than 60 but only 36% for those aged 60 years or older. In this study, the prevalence and severity of tardive dyskinesia increased only up to the age of 70; after that, there was no further increase with advancing age.

Mukherjee et al (1982) examined 153 psychotic outpatients, receiving maintenance doses of neuroleptics, for tardive dyskinesia. Age, but not sex, was found to be significantly correlated with prevalence and severity of the disorder.

Many elderly patients have been taking neuroleptics for longer periods of time than have their younger counterparts. One might consider whether the increased prevalence and severity of tardive dyskinesia among older patients could be explained by their longer exposure to neuroleptics. Perenyi and Arato (1980) studied 200 hospitalized schizophrenic patients, most of whom had received neuroleptic treatment for at least two years, and reported that the frequency and severity of tardive dyskinesia increased with age, and the more advanced the age at which the patient started taking neuroleptics, the more likely it was that tardive dyskinesia would develop. In patients under 30 when therapy with neuroleptics was begun, the incidence of tardive dyskinesia was approximately 18%; in those between 31 and 40 it was 22%; in those between 41 and 50 it was 28%; and in those over 50 it was 50%. Johnson et al (1982) also considered whether the age differences in the prevalence of tardive dyskinesia are artifacts of differential exposure to neuroleptics. They studied 66 patients and, like other authors, reported that the incidence of tardive dyskinesia increased with advancing age. In addition, in their study the severity of tardive dyskinesia also increased with age. In order to distinguish the factor of cumulative dose from age, they separated their patients into four groups (under 33, 34 to 45, 46 to 56, over 57 years of age). They found that the mean length of neuroleptic regimens for the four groups was 2.9, 7.6, 8.3, and 8.4 years, respectively. Apart from the patients aged younger than 33 years, the duration of treatment with neuroleptic drugs does not seem to explain the differences in severity that were found. Unfortunately, Johnson et al presented no data on cumulative neuroleptic doses, but since elderly patients are generally treated with lower doses of neuroleptics than their younger counterparts, it seems unlikely that the elderly patients would have received greater cumulative doses. These findings strongly suggest that the increased prevalence and severity of tardive dyskinesia in older patients cannot be easily explained by longer exposure to neuroleptics.

There is overwhelming evidence that the aging brain is more susceptible to tardive dyskinesia. Studies show that neurotransmitter enzyme synthesis in the basal ganglia decreases with age (Granacher, 1981; McGreer et al, 1977). Some cell loss of dopaminergic tracts has been found with advanced age, but most of the altered enzyme activity seems to be due to decreased function of remaining cells rather than to loss of neurons (McGreer et al, 1977).

Tardive dyskinesia frequently persists after discontinuation of neuroleptic drugs (Uhrbrand and Faurbye, 1960; Rodova and Nahunek, 1964; Hunter et al, 1964; Degwitz et al, 1967; Crane, 1968). This observation has led investigators to search for permanent structural alteration in the brains of patients with tardive dyskinesia (Klawans et al, 1980). Neuropathologic studies following acute or chronic administration of antipsychotic drugs in laboratory animals have not demonstrated specific or localized neuropathologic changes in the brain (Roizin et al, 1959; Julou et al, 1968). There is one report of reduced neuronal cell count in the basal ganglia of rats chronically receiving phenothiazines (Pakkenberg et al, 1972), but this is of uncertain importance because gliosis or degenerative changes were not observed. Postmortem neuropathologic changes in patients after chronic phenothiazine treatment without extrapyramidal movement disorders have usually consisted of scattered areas of neuronal degeneration and gliosis without specific localization (Roizin et al, 1959). Individual patients with drug-induced parkinsonism or tardive dyskinesia have been reported to show, at autopsy, changes in the globus pallidus and putamen (Poursines et al, 1959), in the caudate nucleus and substantia nigra, and in the inferior olive (Gross and Kaltenbach, 1968). Other investigators, however, have reported no significant neuropathologic abnormality in patients with tardive dyskinesia (Hunter et al, 1968).

One study (Christensen et al, 1970) reported the presence of neuronal degeneration and gliosis of the substantia nigra in 27 of 28 brains from patients with chronic oral dyskinesias; 21 of the cases were attributed to antipsychotic drugs. Only seven of 28 matched control brains showed similar changes. Although these changes may represent a toxic effect of the drug, their occurrence in some elderly persons who did not have tardive dyskinesia raises the possibility that they may be events of aging, not directly related to the development of tardive dyskinesia. The fact that no consistent anatomic alterations are associated with tardive dyskinesia has led investigators recently to give more attention to the neurochemistry and pharmacology of the disorder. The pathophysiology of tardive dyskinesia is therefore still unclear, and we have no sure explanation why elderly patients are vulnerable to this disorder.

The best way to prevent tardive dyskinesia is to avoid the use of neuroleptics. Obviously, these drugs are sometimes required, but they should not be used when indications are unclear or when less potentially toxic drugs may be as efficacious. As noted in chapter 1, a recent report (Burke et al, 1982) of 42 patients with tardive dyskinesia seen in movement disorder clinics in London, New York, and Houston found that 19 had been inappropriately treated with neuroleptics. Of these, six patients has been treated for anxiety, six for depression, four for behavioral disturbances associated with mental retardation, and three for an acute psychotic episode precipitated by emotional stress. The therapeutic difficulties, the prolonged and possibly permanent nature of tardive dyskinesia in some cases, and the disability caused by the movements, all serve to emphasize the need to avoid unnecessary use of neuroleptic drugs to treat conditions that can be managed by alternative means.

It is important to make a base-line examination prior to starting neuroleptics and also to recognize the early signs of tardive dyskinesia. They include fine vermicular movements or restlessness of the tongue, mild choreiform finger or toe movements, and facial tics or frequent eye blinks (Gardos and Cole, 1980). Clinical recognition of early tardive dyskinesia involves systematic observation of patients in search for those signs. Crane (1972) recommended examination of drug-maintained patients every three months for signs of tardive dyskinesia. A more aggressive method of detecting the disorder may involve drug holidays for a few days or weeks. A drug-free period of less than three or four weeks is usually too short to precipitate psychotic relapse but long enough to uncover dyskinesia (Gardos and Cole, 1980).

It is important to remember that certain illnesses may cause dyskinesia, and causes of dyskinesias other than tardive dyskinesia should be ruled out. The differential diagnosis of tardive dyskinesia has been reviewed in depth (Granacher, 1981). Indications for neuroleptics should be considered, and suitable alternatives should be tried; for example, lithium carbonate or carbamazepine (Ayd, 1982) for patients with schizoaffective or affective disorders (see chapter 4), benzodiazepines for anxiety (Jenike, 1982a), and propranolol for aggressive or violent patients (Jenike, 1982b; 1983b). In patients known to require antipsychotic drugs, attempts should be made to find the minimal effective dose.

The major classes of drugs used in the treatment of tardive dyskinesia include dopamine antagonists, cholinergic drugs, and γ-aminobutyric acid agonists (Gardos and Cole, 1980; Koboyashi, 1977). None of these has emerged as a satisfactory treatment, but nonspecific measures such as dose reduction may sometimes be helpful in the long term. In view of the significant risk to the elderly patient and the ineffective treatment options, physicians should avoid the use of neuroleptic drugs in elderly patients whenever possible.

Neuroleptic overdose Neuroleptics have a very high therapeutic index (ratio of lethal dose to effective dose) and are unlikely to result in death when taken in large quantities. Patients have survived acute ingestions of many grams of these agents, and it is virtually impossible to commit suicide by an acute overdosage of an antipsychotic agent alone (Baldessarini, 1977). Obviously, when taken in combination with other toxic agents such as alcohol, barbiturates, or tricyclic antidepressants, death may result. Dialysis is not helpful in removing neuroleptics or antidepressants, but can be used to eliminate barbiturates from the body. Physostigmine, a centrally active anticholinesterase agent, can be used to reverse atropinelike anticholinergic symptoms (see chapter 8).

Propranolol

Sometimes violent elderly patients do not respond to large doses of neuroleptics or benzodiazepines. Most of these patients have some type of organic brain disorder and many suffer from dementing illnesses.

Recently, a few case reports suggest that propranolol may be a reasonable alternative (Jenike, 1982b; 1983b). Although the total number of reported cases is small and no controlled studies have been performed yet, there is reason for optimism. At least half of the reported cases in which propranolol produced positive behavioral changes involved elderly demented patients. Petrie and Ban reported on three patients, aged 54, 71, and 86 years, all with the diagnosis of primary dementia (Petrie and Ban, 1981). Although no improvements in memory, cognition, or confusion were noted, propranolol did yield a therapeutic response within two weeks.

The first case was a 54-year-old man with presenile dementia who had a three-year history of progressive personality deterioration. He had been treated with numerous antipsychotics and benzodiazepines, all of which produced disabling side effects, including oversedation and extrapyramidal manifestations. Propranolol, 20 mg three times per day, produced control within two weeks. After a month, when the propranolol was discontinued, the patient promptly relapsed, but remitted after propranolol was resumed.

The second case was a 71-year-old woman with a severe lack of impulse control. Unable to sit still, she intermittently attacked other patients and wandered aimlessly. Haloperidol, up to 20 mg/day, had no therapeutic effect. Following a 10-day course of propranolol in doses of 160 mg/day, the patient showed clear improvement with diminished agitation. She was also able to eat, dress, and communicate more effectively.

The third case involved an 86-year-old woman with a diagnosis of senile dementia. She was unable to care for herself and exhibited rambling, destructive, disorganized behavior. Despite a three-week course of haloperidol, 25 mg/day, she wandered constantly and destroyed furniture, ward furnishings, and even a water fountain. Propranolol, 60 mg/day, rapidly controlled her agitation and destructive behavior.

Yudofsky et al reported four patients with organic brain damage whose violent episodes responded to propranolol (Yudofsky et al, 1981). Three of these patients were young; one had uncontrolled seizures and attacks of rage, another had Wilson's disease, and the third was mentally retarded. The fourth patient was a 63-year-old man who had been struck in the head by an exploding truck tire which resulted in diffuse, prefrontal cortical damage. After awakening from a three-week coma, he remained disoriented, agitated, and episodically violent. He would punch angrily and dangerously at family members and nursing staff while screaming profanities. Antipsychotic medications did little to control his symptoms.

Upon transfer to a neuropsychiatric ward, he became furious, kicking and swinging his fists, and either spitting or shouting curses at staff members. Chlorpromazine, as much as 800 mg/day, was of little value in controlling the recurrent outbursts of rage and violence. Propranolol was administered at dosages up to 80 mg four times per day, and within three weeks the frequency, intensity, and duration of his rage and combativeness were markedly reduced. He was managed at home on 320 mg propranolol and 400 mg chlorpromazine daily. At 26-month follow-up, he had remained at home without rehospitalization.

Greendyke and coworkers (1984) recently reported using up to 520 mg/day of propranolol in eight patients with organic brain disease characterized by violent and assaultive behavior refractory to conventional treatment. Improvement was demonstrated in the seven patients able to tolerate adequate drug dosages.

There are a few other case reports where younger patients with various types of brain injuries responded similarly to propranolol (Mansheim, 1981; Schreier, 1979; Elliott, 1977). However, there appear to be no reports in the literature where non-brain–damaged patients exhibiting rage and violent tendencies were helped by the administration of propranolol.

In the case studies described above, bradycardia and hypotension were the most common side effects of propranolol. Propranolol can cause myocardial depression, which can lead to congestive heart failure. Vital signs should be monitored frequently, particularly during the early phases of treatment and when dosage is being increased (*AMA Drug Evaluations,* 1980). Propranolol is contrindicated in most patients with congestive heart failure; patients receiving most types of general anesthesia; patients with bronchial asthma or allergic or nonallergic bronchospasm (ie, emphysema); patients with a severe sinus bradycardia; patients with ventricular failure or in cardiogenic shock; and many insulin-dependent diabetics and those prone to hypoglycemia (Yudofsky et al, 1981).

The mechanism by which propranolol exerts its effects on violent behavior in elderly patients is unknown at present. It is lipid-soluble, and thus passes through the blood-brain barrier; it also acts peripherally on β-adrenergic receptors (Sheppard, 1979). Researchers speculate that it either acts on the brain to somehow mitigate the disinhibition of the response to rage caused by CNS lesions, or on the peripheral nervous system as a β-blocker to reduce somatic responses to frustration, fear, or panic that may trigger outbursts of rage (Yudofsky et al, 1981; Heiser and DeFrancisco, 1976; Cole et al, 1979).

Although propranolol has not been approved by the Food and Drug Administration for any psychiatric illness, possible psychiatric implications have been explored worldwide for more than 15 years (Cole et al, 1979; Ayd, 1981). The use of propranolol for an unapproved indication is not illegal, but it would be wise to advise patients and their families that it is an innovative form of therapy. Both the discussion with the patient and family and the rationale for using propranolol should be documented in the medical record (Gelenberg, 1981).

In summary, even though mechanisms remain speculative, it is clinically important to note that the severely disabling rage and belligerent behavior of some previously unmanageable patients with CNS lesions or disease have been controlled by the use of high doses of propranolol. In the cases reported thus far, a therapeutic response was noted between ten days and three weeks, with doses ranging from 60 to 550 mg/day. There was no improvement in cognition, confusion levels, or memory proficiency with the use of propranolol in any of these patients.

Carbamazepine

There is some evidence that carbamazepine (Tegretol) may be helpful in treating some elderly patients who exhibit severely disabling rage and belligerent behavior. There have been two recent reports indicating that carbamazepine might be useful in the treatment of psychiatric patients who have EEG abnormalities (Hakola and Laulumaa, 1982; Neppe, 1983). From these reports, however, it was not clear if this drug would help similar patients who had normal EEGs. To address this question, Luchins (1983) studied violent patients on two long-stay psychiatric wards who had received carbamazepine for at least six weeks as an adjunct to neuroleptics. All of these patients had a normal EEG (while off carbamazepine and without nasopharyngeal leads) and did not have affective disorder. Luchins ruled out affective disorder since it was already known that such patients may respond to carbamazepine in the absence of an EEG abnormality (Post, 1982) (see chapter 4). Luchins found seven patients (five males); six were diagnosed as schizophrenic and the other had a mixed personality disorder (DSM III criteria). He retrospectively reviewed nursing notes of episodes of physical aggression during the periods when these patients were on and off carbamazepine. All were on carbamazepine for a period of time; then it was discontinued for a six-week period, and then begun again. The mean number of aggressive episodes while taking carbamazepine was significantly less than either before or after drug treatment. Six of the seven patients had fewer aggressive episodes during the carbamazepine period than either before or after. All patients were receiving neuroleptics throughout the period of this study and there was no difference in the mean neuroleptic dosage either before, during, or after carbamazepine administration. The mean carbamazepine dosage was 1057 mg/day (range 400 to 1600 mg) with a mean serum concentration of 8.5 μg/mL (range 6.3 to 13 μg/mL).

Luchin's findings need to be confirmed in a double-blind controlled trial. Furthermore, one cannot rule out the possibility that more extensive EEG studies would have detected an abnormality in these patients. Nevertheless, these cases do suggest that a normal clinical EEG in a violent elderly patient may not preclude a beneficial response to carbamazepine. In addition, these findings raise the possibility that carbamazepine's psychotropic effects may not be related to its anticonvulsive action. Moreover, since the drug's spectrum of psychotropic effects parallels that of lithium, with both being useful in agressive patients (Sheard, 1975) as well as in the treatment and prophylaxis of affective disorders (Post, 1982), it would seem likely that some mechanism common to both drugs underlies their shared effects.

Even though none of the patients in Luchin's study suffered from dementia, carbamazepine may be a reasonable drug to try in the demented patient where other agents have not been useful in controlling violent or aggressive behavior.

Lithium Carbonate

Since its introduction by Cade in 1949, lithium carbonate has become widely accepted as a treatment for manic-depressive illness (Cade, 1949; Sheard, 1975). Lithium is very effective at controlling hyperaggressiveness and hypersexuality, frequent concomitants of manic-depressive episodes. Lithium also plays an inhibitory role in animal aggressive behavior including that induced by hypthalamic stimulation in cats (Wasman and Flynn, 1972). In epileptic patients, lithium has reportedly produced interseizure behavioral improvements in patients who were impulsive, excited, and aggressive (Gershon and Trantner, 1956; Gershon 1968; Glesinger, 1954; Williamson, 1966). On the other hand, one study (Jus et al, 1973) of 18 female patients with temporal lobe epilepsy showed that lithium worsened seizure activity. Other reports confirm that lithium may induce grand mal seizures (Sheard, 1975) and thus the effect of lithium on convulsive disorders is still debated.

In brain damaged children with periodic aggression (Annell, 1969), and in severely mentally retarded adolescents (Dostal and Zvoltsky, 1970), lithium reportedly has antiaggressive effects.

There are two reported trials of lithium in man where abnormal aggressive behavior was the predominant manifestation and source of difficulty (Sheard, 1975). One studied 12 chronically assaultive males with lithium versus placebo in a single-blind cross-over trial. None of the subjects had overt evidence of brain damage or psychosis and all had IQs over 85. Lithium was maintained at blood levels of 0.8 to 1.2 mEq/L for 1 month, then 1 month of placebo, and finally another month of lithium was given. There was a significant reduction in aggressive incidents in lithium periods as compared to placebo (Sheard, 1971). The second study (Tupin et al, 1973) confirmed these findings in a longer trial involving 27 violent male convicts who were treated for up to 18 months with lithium carbonate. Again, there was a significant reduction in the number of violent incidents as compared with the number in the same length of time before treatment began. Many of these convicts were diagnosed as schizophrenic and some had brain damage.

There are no controlled trials of lithium in elderly brain-damaged patients who are violent. Lithium should be tried if other measures fail. Lithium is clearly indicated in elderly patients with pre-existing manic-depressive illness (see chapter 4).

SUMMARY

Violent, psychotic, or aggressive elderly patients are among the most difficult patients to manage. A number of medications are helpful to the clinician faced with such a patient. Neuroleptics are the mainstay of treatment but have many potentially disabling side effects. They should be used in the lowest possible dose to minimize unwanted effects. Haloperidol in doses of 0.5 mg twice daily or thiothixene 1 mg twice daily are reasonable starting doses. In the very frail elderly, doses as low as 0.25 mg of haloperidol at bedtime may have a therapeutic effect.

Low-potency agents, such as chlorpromazine and thioridazine, have more associated sedation, orthostatic hypotension, anticholinergic effects, and cardiovascular problems, but have fewer extrapyramidal effects than the high-potency agents. For this reason, they are preferred in patients with pre-existing movement disorders such as Parkinson's disease. Doses as low as 10 mg twice daily should be tried initially.

Neuroleptic side effects have been reviewed and the use of alternate medications such as propranolol, carbamazepine, and lithium carbonate are discussed. Neuroleptics should be avoided whenever possible. Indications for neuroleptic treatment should be reviewed periodically so that patients are exposed to risks and side effects for the minimum possible duration.

REFERENCES

AMA Drug Evaluations, ed 4. Chicago, American Medical Association, 1980, pp 533–535.

Annell AL: Lithium in the treatment of children and adolescents. *Acta Psychiatr Scand Suppl* 207:19–33, 1969.

Ayd FJ: Carbamazepine's acute and prophylactic effects in manic and depressive illness: An update. *Int Drug Ther Newsletter* 17:2,3,5, 1982.

Ayd FJ: Propranolol for rage and violence. *Int Drug Ther Newsletter* 16:19–20, 1981.

Baldessarini RJ: *Chemotherapy in Psychiatry*. Cambridge, Mass, Harvard University Press, 1977.

Bartter FC: *The Syndrome of Inappropriate Secretion of Antidiuretic Hormone*. Chicago, Year Book Medical Publishers, 1973.

Bernstein JG: Chemotherapy of psychosis, in Bernstein JG (ed): *Clinical Psychopharmacology*. Littleton, Mass, PSG Publishing Co Inc, 1978, pp 40–51.

Burke RE, Fahn S, Janovic J, et al: Tardive dyskinesia and inappropriate use of neuroleptic drugs. *Lancet* 1:1299, 1982.

Cade JFJ: Lithium salts in the treatment of psychotic excitement. *Med J Aust* 36:349–352, 1949.

Christensen E, Moller JE, Faurbye A: Neuropathological investigation of 28 brains from patients with dyskinesias. *Acta Psychiatr Scand* 46:14, 1970.

Cole JO, Altesman RI, Weingarten CH: Beta-blocking drugs in psychiatry. *McLean Hosp J* 4:40–68, 1979.

Crane GE: Tardive dyskinesia in patients treated with neuroleptics: A review of the literature. *Am J Psychiatry* 124 (February Suppl):4O, 1968.

Crane GE. Prevention and management of tardive dyskinesia. *Am J Psychiatry* 129:781, 1972.

Davies P: Neurotransmitter-related symptoms in SDAT. *Brain Res* 171:319, 1979.

Degwitz R, Binsack KF, Herkert H: Zur Problem der persistierenden extrapyramidelen Hyperkinesen nach langfristiger Anwendung von Neuroleptica. *Nervenarzt* 38:170, 1967.

DiMascio A, Bernardo DL, Greenblatt DJ, et al: A controlled trial of amantadine in drug-induced extrapyramidal disorders. *Arch Gen Psychiatry* 33:599–602, 1976.

Dostal T, Zvoltsky P: Antiaggressive effect of lithium salts in several mentally retarded adolescents. *Int Pharmacopsychiatry* 5:203–207, 1970.

Drachman DA, Leavitt J: Human memory and the cholinergic system. *Arch Neurol* 30:113–121, 1974.

Ekbom KA: Asthenia crurum paresthesia (irritable legs). *Acta Med Scand* 118:197, 1944.

Ekbom KA: Restless legs and akathisia. *J Swedish Med Assoc* 62:2376–2382, 1965.

Elliott FA: Propranolol for the control of belligerent behavior following acute brain damage. *Ann Neurol* 1:489–491, 1977.

Gardos G, Cole JO: Overview: Public health issues in tardive dyskinesia. *Am J Psychiatry* 137:776, 1980.

Gelenberg AJ: Treating the outpatient schizophrenic. *Postgrad Med* 64:48–55, 1978.

Gelenberg AJ: The long arm of propranolol: Extension to organic mental disorders. *Biological Therapies in Psychiatry* 4:13–14, 1981.

Gershon S: The use of lithium salts in psychiatric disorders. *Dis Nerv Syst* 29:51–62, 1968.

Gershon S, Trantner EM: The treatment of shock dependency by pharmacological agents. *Med J Aust* 43:783–787, 1956.

Glesinger B: Evaluation of lithium in the treatment of psychotic excitement. *Med J Aust* 41:277–283, 1954.

Granacher RP: Differential diagnosis of tardive dyskinesia: An overview. *Am J Psychiatry* 138:1288, 1981.

Greendyke RM, Schuster DB, Wooten JA: Propranolol in the treatment of assaultive patients with organic brain disease. *J Clin Psychopharmacol* 4:282–285, 1984.

Gross H, Kaltenback E: Neuropathological findings in persistent dyskinesia after neuroleptic long term therapy, in Cerlett A, Boue FJ (eds): *The Present Status of Psychotropic Drugs.* Amsterdam, Excerpta Medica, 1968.

Hakola HPA, Laulumaa BAO: Carbamazepine in treatment of violent schizophrenics. *Lancet* 1:1358, 1982.

Heiser JF, DeFrancisco D: The treatment of pathological panic states with propranolol. *Am J Psychiatry* 133:1389–1394, 1976.

Hunter R, Earl CJ, Janz D: A syndrome of abnormal movements and dementia in leukotomized patients treated with phenothiazines. *J Neurol Neurosurg Psychiatry* 27:219, 1964.

Hunter R, Blackwood W, Smith MC, et al: Neuropathological findings in 3 cases of persistent dyskinesias following phenothiazine medication. *J Neurol Sci* 7:763, 1968.

Husband C, Mal FM, Carruthers G: Syndrome of inappropriate secretion of antidiuretic hormone in a patient treated with haloperidol. *Can J Psychiatry* 26:197–197, 1981.

Jenike MA: Using sedative drugs in the elderly. *Drug Therapy* 12:184–190, 1982a.

36

Jenike MA: Propranolol as treatment of rage and violence in elderly patients. *Topics in Geriatrics* 1:5–60, 1982b.

Jenike MA: Tardive dyskinesia: Special risk in the elderly. *J Am Geriatr Soc* 31:71–73, 1983a.

Jenike MA: Treatment of rage and violence in elderly patients with propranolol. *Geriatrics* 38:29–34, 1983b.

Johnson GFS, Hunt GE, Rey JM: Incidence and severity of tardive dyskinesia with age. *Arch Gen Psychiatry* 39:486, 1982.

Julou L, Ducrot R, Ganter P, et al: Chronic toxicity, side effects and metabolism of neuroleptics of the phenothiazine group, in *Proceedings of the European Society for Study of Drug Toxicity*. Amsterdam, Excerpta Medica, 1968, vol. 9: *Toxicity and Side Effects of Psychotropic Drugs, International Congress Series 145*.

Jus A, Villeneuve A, Goutier J, et al: Some remarks on the influence of lithium carbonate on patients with temporal epilepsy. *Int J Clin Pharmacol Ther Toxicol* 7:67–74, 1973.

Kane JM, Smith JM: Tardive dyskinesia. *Arch Gen Psychiatry* 39:473, 1982.

Klawans HL, Goetz CG, Perliks S: Tardive dyskinesia: Review and update. *Am J Psychiatry* 137:900, 1980.

Kobayashi RM: Drug therapy of tardive dyskinesia. *N Engl J Med* 296:259, 1977.

Lipinski JF, Zubenko GS, Cohen BM, et al: Propranolol and the treatment of neuroleptic-induced akathisia. *Am J Psychiatry* 141:412–415, 1984.

Luchins DJ: Carbamazepine for the violent psychiatric patient. *Lancet* 1:766, 1983.

Mansheim P: Treatment with propranolol of the behavioral sequelae of brain damage. *J Clin Psychiatry* 42:132, 1981.

Matuk F, Kalyanaraman K: Syndrome of inappropriate secretion of antidiuretic hormone in patients treated with psychotropic drugs. *Arch Neurol* 34:375–375, 1977.

McGreer PL, McGreer EG, Suzoki JS: Aging and extrapyramidal function. *Arch Neurol* 34:33, 1977.

Miller M, Moses AM: Drug-induced states of impaired water excretion. *Kidney Int* 10:96–103, 1976.

Mukherjee S, Rosen AM, Cardemas C, et al: Tardive dyskinesia in psychiatric outpatients. *Arch Gen Psychiatry* 39:466, 1982.

Neppe VM: Carbamazepine in the psychiatric outpatient. *Lancet* 1:766, 1983.

Pakkenberg H, Fog R, Nilakantan B: The long term effect of perphenazine enanthate on the rat brain: Some metabolic and anatomical observations. *Psychopharmacologia* 29:329, 1972.

Perenyi A, Arato M: Tardive dyskinesia on Hungarian psychiatric wards. *Psychosomatics* 21:904, 1980.

Petrie WM, Ban TA: Propranolol in organic agitation. *Lancet* 1:324, 1981.

Post RM: Use of the anticonvulsant carbamazepine in primary and secondary affective illness: Clinical and theoretical implications. *Psychol Med* 12:701–704, 1982.

Poursines Y, Alliez J, Toga M: Syndrome parkinsonien consecutif a la prise prolongee de chlorpromazine avec ictus mortel intercurrent. *Rev Neurol (Paris)* 100:745, 1959.

Rao KJ, Miller M, Moses A: Water intoxication and thioridazine (Mellaril). *Ann Intern Med* 82:61, 1975.

Raskind M: Psychosis, polydipsia and water intoxication. *Arch Gen Psychiatry* 30:112–114, 1974.

Rivera JLGD: Inappropriate secretion of antidiuretic hormone from fluphenazine therapy. *Ann Intern Med* 82:811–812, 1975.

Rodova A, Nahunek R: Persistent dyskinesia after phenothiazines. *Cesk Psychiatr* 60:250, 1964.

Roizin L, True C, Kuigut M: Structural effects of tranquilizers. *Res Publ Assoc Res Nerv Ment Dis* 37:285, 1959.

Schreier HA: Use of propranolol in the treatment of postencephalitic psychosis. *Am J Psychiatry* 136:840–841, 1979.

Sheard MH: Effect of lithium in human aggression. *Nature* 230:113–114, 1971.

Sheard MH: Lithium in the treatment of aggression. *J Nerv Ment Dis* 160:108–118, 1975.

Sheppard GP: High dose propranolol in schizophrenia. *Br J Psychiatry* 134:470–476, 1979.

Smith JM, Baldessarini RJ: Changes in prevalence, severity, and recovery in tardive dyskinesia with age. *Arch Gen Psychiatry* 37:1368, 1980.

Snyder SH, Banerjee SP, Yamamura HI, et al: Drugs, neurotransmitters and schizophrenia. *Science* 184:1234–1253, 1974.

Sos J, Cassem NH: Intravenous use of haloperidol for acute delirium in intensive care settings, in Speidel H, Rodewald G (eds): *Psychic and Neurological Dysfunctions After Open-Heart Surgery*. Stuttgart, Georg Thieme Verlag, 1980, pp 196–199.

Spira N, Dysken MW, Lazarus LW, et al: Treatment of agitation and psychosis, in Salzman C (ed): *Clinical Geriatric Psychopharmacology*. New York, McGraw-Hill Book Co, 1984, pp 49–76.

Strang RR: The symptoms of restless legs. *Med J Aust* 1(24):1211–1213, 1967.

Tupin JP, Smith DB, Classon TL, et al: Long-term use of lithium in aggressive prisoners. *Compr Psychiatry* 14:311–317, 1973.

Uhrbrand L, Faurbye A: Reversible and irreversible dyskinesia after treatment with perphenazine, chlorpromazine, reserpine, ECT therapy. *Psychopharmacologia* 1:408, 1960.

Van Putten T, Mutalipassi LR, Malkin MD: Phenothiazine-induced decompensation. *Arch Gen Psychiatry* 30:102–105, 1974.

Van Putten T: The many faces of akathisia. *Compr Psychiatry* 16:43–47, 1975.

Wasman M, Flynn JP: Direct attack elicited from hypothalamus. *Arch Neurol* 6:220–227, 1972.

Williamson B: Psychiatry since lithium. *Dis Nerv Syst* 27:775–782, 1966.

Yudofsky S, Williams D, Gorman J: Propranolol in the treatment of rage and violent behavior in patients with chronic brain syndrome. *Am J Psychiatry* 138:218–220, 1981.

*"Aging is when the best part of your day is over when
your alarm clock goes off."*

CHAPTER 4

Affective Illness

Loss, sadness, and grief are common experiences of old age. Depression, however, is a life-threatening disorder that may affect nearly a million older Americans. In some studies of community-dwelling elderly citizens, the prevalence of clinical depression has been reported as high as 13% (Gurland, 1976). As many as 20% to 35% of elderly patients with concurrent medical illness are depressed (Anonymous, 1979; Moffie and Paykel, 1975). Those over age 65 account for about 11% of the US population, but commit about 25% of all suicides (Sendbuehler and Goldstein, 1977). In addition, a number of studies have demonstrated that untreated major depression lowers life expectancy and is associated with a greater risk for cardiac disease (Kay and Bergman, 1966; Avery and Winokur, 1976; Tsuang et al, 1980). Depressed elderly patients are often malnourished and agitated for months or even years (Jefferson and Marshall, 1981). In view of the effective therapies available for depression, it is especially crucial to make the diagnosis and proceed with treatment (Jenike, 1983a).

RECOGNIZING DEPRESSION

It is not always easy to diagnose depression in the elderly, who may present with various clinical pictures such as chronic pain, multiple somatic complaints, or even the picture of dementia (pseudodementia). Depression is, in fact, the main cause of a treatable dementia in the elderly (Wells, 1963; Feinberg and Goodman, 1984; Cole et al, 1983).

Although some elderly depressed individuals present atypically, most can be diagnosed according to the Washington University research criteria, which form the basis for the DSM-III criteria (Spar and LaRue, 1983). A helpful mnemonic, developed by Dr Carey Gross at Massachusetts General Hospital, that outlines the clinical picture of depression is SIG E CAPS: *S*leep, *I*nterest, *G*uilt, *E*nergy, *C*oncentration, *A*ppetite, *P*sychomotor, and *S*uicide (Figure 4-1). Each of these corresponds to one of the DSM-III criteria for Major Depression (Jenike, 1983b; Jenike, 1984a). To elaborate, depressed patients generally complain of insomnia, typically with early awakening in the morning; occasionally, however, hypersomnia is the problem. They lose interest in usually stimulating activities — job, hobbies, social activities, and sex. Guilty ruminations and feelings of self-reproach are the rule. Depressed patients have no energy and feel fatigued all day. They frequently report an inability to concentrate, with slowed or mixed-up thinking. They usually have a poor appetite with an associated loss of weight, although occasionally they overeat. Psychomotor retardation is usually observed, but agitated depressions in the elderly are not uncommon. They may have recurrent thoughts of suicide or death and may feel that life is not worth living or wish that they were dead. A patient with at least four of these eight criteria is depressed and if his dysphoric emotional state has persisted for two to four weeks, he needs treatment.

Another clue to recognizing depression is the presence of multiple

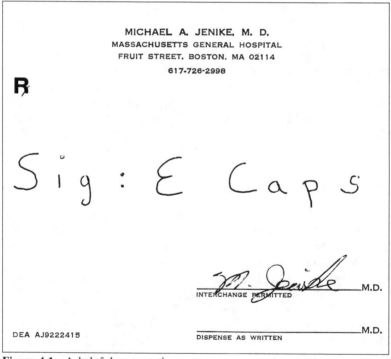

Figure 4-1 A helpful mnemonic.

complaints in several body systems. When a patient's complaints do not fit a recognizable pattern or when chronic pain is a component, depression should be suspected and the SIG E CAPS criteria should be investigated. When elderly patients appear demented, special care is required to rule out depression (see chapter 6). Initially, family members should be asked if they have observed any of the SIG E CAPS symptoms in the patient. There are a few clinical points that are helpful in the differentiation between depression and dementia (Wells, 1963). The onset of Alzheimer's dementia is typically insidious, whereas the beginning of endogenous depression with pseudodementia is more often acute and recent. A careful history may reveal that cognitive impairment was not evident until the onset of depressive symptoms in pseudodementia. A demented patient may be affectively shallow, although this is not invariably the case; whereas a depressed patient is often upset with his condition. If there is any doubt whether a patient is depressed, he should be treated. Many patients are both demented and depressed and the only way to clearly separate the two components is by their response to treatment. Depression, even in a patient with an underlying dementing process, can usually be resolved. Cognition may not improve but patients will become less negative, more interested in hobbies and sex, and family members frequently will report dramatic improvement in the patient's mood and outlook on life.

DIFFERENTIAL DIAGNOSIS

When it has been determined that a patient is depressed, it is necessary to rule out both medical and psychiatric causes. Some psychiatric conditions that can include depression are manic-depressive disease, schizophrenia, psychotic depression, borderline personality disorder, alcoholism, and unresolved grief (Jenike and Anderson, 1984).

In manic-depressive disorders, the depressive state is indistinguishable from other types of depression and a history of a previous manic episode in the patient or in his family is the key to diagnosis.

A schizophrenic may appear depressed but at some time will have delusions, hallucinations, or a thought disorder. Hallucinations are characteristically auditory (visual hallucinations suggest a medical cause) and the patient may believe that others can hear what he is thinking (thought broadcasting) or that they are putting thoughts or ideas into his head (thought insertion). Ideas of reference (eg, television or radio communicating about him or talking to him directly) and paranoia are common.

Some alcoholics have a primary affective disorder that they are attempting to treat by drinking. A careful alcohol history is mandatory in depressed patients.

Grieving patients may appear depressed and they frequently experience a syndrome of shortness of breath, frequent sighing, an empty feeling in the abdomen, lack of muscular strength, and extreme tension (Lazare, 1979). Often they feel that every task is a major effort and that life has no meaning. Sometimes the bereaved takes on the traits of the deceased or the symptoms of his last illness. Uncomplicated grief may last six months or more. In one study, 17% of bereaved persons were clinically depressed one year after the death of a spouse or close family member (Clayton, 1974).

When taking the history the physician should inquire about recent illnesses and operations, mental status changes, and current drug and medication use. The patient's support systems — the availability and reliability of family or friends — should be evaluated. Psychiatric syndromes causing depression can easily be eliminated from the differential diagnosis by asking about prior manic or psychotic episodes, present disturbing thoughts, recent deaths of people close to the patient, and alcohol use.

Many physical illnesses may be associated with depression and should be considered in the workup of all depressed patients (Table 4-1) (Anderson, 1979; Jenike and Anderson, 1984). Although it is clearly impractical to rule out all potential causes of depression, the physician must look for certain life-threatening conditions. These include diuretic-induced hypokalemia or hyponatremia, Addison's disease, hypoparathyroidism, severe anemia, pneumonia, myocardial infarction, congestive heart failure, uremia, hepatic encephalopathy, Wernicke's encephalopathy, meningitis, and encephalitis.

All depressed elderly patients must have a physical examiniation, mental status examination, and basic laboratory tests including a complete blood count with differential and electrolyte determinations to identify any life-threatening conditions (Jenike, 1984a). Once potentially disastrous physical illnesses have been eliminated, the physician's primary concern is deciding who will treat the patient and how the patient will be treated.

SUICIDAL ASSESSMENT

Studies consistently reveal that about 15% of the total deaths of patients with affective disorder are due to suicides (Avery and Winokur, 1976). The physician must evaluate the possibility that the patient will commit suicide. There is a common fear that asking a depressed person

Table 4-1
Medical Causes of Depression

Deficiency States	*Malignant Disease*
Pellagra	Metastases
Pernicious anemia	Breast
Wernicke's encephalopathy	GI
	Lung
Drugs and Medication	Pancreas
Alcohol	Prostate
Amphetamines	Remote effect: pancreas
Antihypertensive agents	
Clonidine	*Metabolic disorders*
Diuretics—hypokalemia*	Electrolyte imbalance
or hyponatremia*	Hypokalemia
Guanethidine	Hyponatremia
Methyldopa	Hepatic encephalopathy
Propranolol	Hypo-oxygenation
Reserpine	Cerebral arteriosclerosis
Birth control pills	Chronic bronchitis
Cimetidine	Congestive heart failure*
Digitalis	Emphysema
Disulfiram	Myocardial infarction*
Sedatives	Paroxysmal dysrhythmias
Barbiturates	Pneumonia*
Benzodiazepines	Severe anemia*
Steroids/ACTH	Uremia*
Endocrine Disorders	*Neurologic Disorders*
Acromegaly	Alzheimer's disease
Adrenal	Amyotrophic lateral sclerosis
Addison's disease*	Creutzfeldt-Jakob disease
Cushing's disease	Huntington's chorea
Hyper- and hypoparathyroidism*	Multiple sclerosis
Hyper- and hypothyroidism	Myasthenia gravis
Insulinoma	Normal-pressure hydrocephalus
Pheochromocytoma	Parkinson's disease
Pituitary	Pick's disease
	Wilson's disease
Infections	
Encephalitis	*Trauma*
Fungal	Postconcussion
Meningitis	
Neurosyphilis	
Tuberculosis	

*Acute life-threatening disorders.
Reproduced with permission from: Jenike MA: Depressed in the E.R. *Emergency Med* 16:102-120, 1984.

about suicide will plant the idea in his mind or precipitate an attempt. This is not the case and, in fact, patients are generally relieved when the topic is brought up and are surprisingly open about their thoughts and plans. Not asking about suicidal ideation can be a fatal mistake (Jenike, 1984a).

The history can be very helpful. The suicide rate peaks for men between the ages of 80 and 90 and for women between 50 and 65 (Resnick and Cantor, 1967). Alcohol abusers are prone to suicide. A sudden calm in a previously depressed suicidal patient may indicate a definite resolve to die. A psychiatric history or previous attempt increases the likelihood of suicide, as does the presence of physical illness. A psychotic depressed patient is at great risk of suicide, especially if he is hearing voices commanding him to hurt himself. Patients who live alone who perceive themselves as without friends or social support systems are more prone to suicide than those who feel loved.

If there is a serious potential for suicide or if a patient is in a high-risk category, he/she should be hospitalized for protection and further evaluation. Hospitalization is mandatory for a psychotic patient who is talking about suicide, has command hallucinations to hurt himself, or has tried to hurt himself, even if the attempt was trivial; for a survivor of a near-lethal, violent, or premeditated suicide attempt; and for a survivor of a suicide attempt in which there was little chance of rescue. Hospitalization should be considered for a patient who seems unable to care for himself and has no one to care for him, for a survivor of a trivial suicidal attempt who regrets having survived or refuses help, and for a patient who lives alone.

If the patient is intoxicated with drugs or alcohol as well as depressed or suicidal, it is wisest to keep him in a quiet area, with restraints if necessary. His suicide potential and depression can then be evaluated when he is no longer intoxicated. If this is not feasible, a brief hospitalization is necessary. In one study of over 300 patients who were seen in an emergency room after an unsuccessful suicide attempt, 67% of the patients went home the same day, 11% either ran away or signed out against medical advice, and only 17% were sent to a psychiatric unit (Guggenheim, 1978). The overwhelming majority of patients discharged after attempting suicide were still alive at the end of one year. Despite these figures, it is best to err on the side of conservatism when dealing with a suicidal patient. As with appendectomy, a certain number of false-positives is to be expected with optimal medical care. Such patients will probably be released within a few days if an extended evaluation indicates that hospitalization is unwarranted.

If the risk of suicide seems low, the patient need not be hospitalized. Many depressed patients are not thinking clearly and need directed assistance. Such patients will feel a sense of hopelessness but the physician should convey a feeling of optimism.

THE DEXAMETHASONE SUPPRESSION TEST

Not only is depression a common finding in the elderly, but, as mentioned earlier, it is also frequently characterized by atypical presentations which hinder the clinician's ability to make the diagnosis. In recent years, much has been written about the use of the dexamethasone suppression test (DST) as a clinical aid in the evaluation of depressed individuals (Jenike, 1982a; 1982b; 1983c).

Rationale and Procedure for the DST

Normally, plasma cortisol levels fluctuate in a diurnal pattern with maximal levels of up to 25 μg/dL around 6 AM and minimal levels below 8 μg/dL around midnight (Martin et al, 1977). Dexamethasone is a potent glucocorticoid, which suppresses endogenous ACTH and cortisol production for up to 24 hours in normal subjects. The DST is administered as follows. Day 1: At 11 PM 1 mg of dexamethasone is given orally. Day 2: At 8 AM, 4 PM, and 11 PM, blood is drawn for serum cortisol determinations.

The test basically involves serum cortisol sampling after a dose of dexamethasone to see if cortisol levels have been suppressed. DST results are considered abnormal if any of the postdexamethasone serum cortisol levels exceed 5 μg/dL (Carroll et al, 1981). It may not always be possible to draw blood three times on day 2, particularly for outpatients. It has, however, been demonstrated that about 98% of abnormal test results can be obtained by only the 4 PM and 11 PM samples. With the 4 PM sample alone, almost 80% of nonsuppressors (abnormal DST) will be detected (Brown, 1981).

DST abnormalities imply the existence of hypothalamic imbalance and, in addition, clinical manifestations of depressive illness typically include several symptoms that suggest hypothalamic dysfunction, namely, disturbances of mood, sex drive, appetite, sleep, and autonomic activity with frequent diurnal variation in symptoms. Also, the same neurotransmitters implicated in the chemical pathology of depressive illness, particularly serotonin and norepinephrine, have been shown to regulate the secretion of hypothalamic hormones (Sachar et al, 1980). The physiology of the hypothalamic-pituitary-adrenal axis has been well studied. Plasma cortisol levels reflect limbic, hypothalamic, pituitary, and adrenal gland interactions (Kalin et al, 1981). The hypothalamus secretes corticotropin releasing factor (CRF) in response to limbic commands mediated through stimulatory pathways, which are either cholinergic or serotonergic, and adrenergic inhibitory pathways (Jenike, 1982b). CRF is transported via the pituitary portal vasculature to the anterior lobe of the pituitary gland, which stimulates the release of adrenocorticotropic hormone (ACTH), which, in turn, causes secretion of cortisol from the adrenal gland. Cortisol regulates the activity of the system by negative feedback on both the pituitary and hypothalamus (Figure 4-2).

Applications

The DST has been used by endocrinologists for many years to aid in the diagnosis of disorders such as Cushing's syndrome. More recently, however, there has been mounting evidence that the DST is useful as an indicator of hypothalamic-pituitary-adrenal axis abnormalities associated with depressive illness (Carroll et al, 1981). Early researchers noted that cortisol levels were elevated and ACTH secretion disregulated in many depressed patients (Gelenberg, 1983).

Until recently, it appeared that psychiatric disorders other than depression, such as schizophrenia and manic-depressive illness, were not associated with cortisol nonsuppression after dexamethasone administration (Schlesser et al, 1980). Some recent reports, however, suggest that a positive DST may not be as specific to depression as originally thought. Two groups have reported high percentages of abnormal DSTs among manic patients (Graham et al, 1982; Arana et al, 1983) and another set of researchers found positive DSTs in as many as 30% of apparently nondepressed, nonmelancholic, chronic schizophrenic patients (Dewan et al, 1982). Others report that patients with primary obsessive-compulsive disorder had an abnormal DST response (Insel et al, 1982). Many of these patients were concomitantly depressed and supporters of the DST would argue that depression produced the abnormal DST results and not primarily the mania, schizophrenia, or obsessive-compulsive disorder. However one interprets the data, it is clear that the DST is not a definitive biochemical marker for depression. It may, in fact, turn out to be more analogous to an ESR. That is, it could indicate pathology of the neuroendocrine system and must be combined with the entire clinical picture to assist in making the diagnosis. Also, as with the ESR, it may be a useful marker to follow the course and resolution of psychiatric disease processes.

Certain medical conditions and medication use must be eliminated

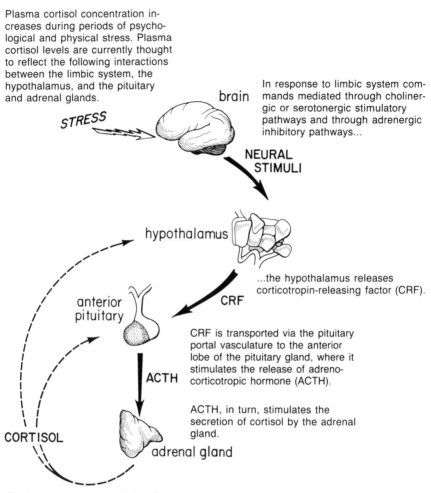

Plasma cortisol concentration increases during periods of psychological and physical stress. Plasma cortisol levels are currently thought to reflect the following interactions between the limbic system, the hypothalamus, and the pituitary and adrenal glands.

STRESS

brain

In response to limbic system commands mediated through cholinergic or serotonergic stimulatory pathways and through adrenergic inhibitory pathways...

NEURAL STIMULI

hypothalamus

...the hypothalamus releases corticotropin-releasing factor (CRF).

anterior pituitary

CRF

CRF is transported via the pituitary portal vasculature to the anterior lobe of the pituitary gland, where it stimulates the release of adrenocorticotropic hormone (ACTH).

ACTH

ACTH, in turn, stimulates the secretion of cortisol by the adrenal gland.

CORTISOL

adrenal gland

Cortisol regulates the activity of this system through negative feedback (---->) to both the pituitary and the hypothalamus.

Figure 4-2 Physiologic basis for the dexamethasone suppression test. Adapted from Jenike MA: Dexamethasone suppression: A biological marker of depression. *Drug Therapy* 9:203-212, 1982.

as a cause of an abnormal DST result in the depressed patient. Conditions that may produce an abnormal DST include alcoholism (during and after withdrawal) (Rees et al, 1977; Oxenkrug, 1978), anorexia nervosa (Carroll, 1978), prolonged hemodialysis (McDonald et al, 1979;

Wallace et al, 1980), Cushing's syndrome (Kalin et al, 1981), malignancies with ectopic ACTH secretion (mostly small cell bronchogenic carcinoma) (Martin et al, 1977), obesity (Streeten et al, 1969) protein-calorie malnutrition (Smith et al, 1975), renovascular hypertension (Cade et al, 1976), and uncontrolled diabetes mellitus (Carroll et al, 1981). Some medications enhance dexamethasone suppression: high-dose benzodiazepines (Carroll, 1972), corticosteroids (including topical and nasal preparations) (Michael et al, 1967), and dextroamphetamine (Sachar et al, 1981). Other drugs cause a lack of dexamethasone suppression by stimulating hepatic metabolism and decreasing dexamethasone half-life: phenytoin (Carroll et al, 1981; Jukiz et al, 1970), barbiturates (Carroll et al, 1981; Brooks et al, 1972), and meprobamate (Carroll et al, 1981). Alcohol produces an apparent lack of dexamethasone suppression by increasing plasma cortisol (Elias and Gwinup, 1980). L-tryptophan is known to enhance central serotonin and has an uncertain effect on the DST (Nuller and Ostroumova, 1980). Interestingly, most psychotropic drugs, including neuroleptics, tricyclic antidepressants, MAOIs and lithium carbonate, do not affect the DST (Schlesser et al, 1980; Carroll et al, 1976; Brown et al, 1979; Amsterdam et al, 1982).

The three-sample DST can reportedly identify depressed patients with a sensitivity of 67% and a specificity of 96% (Carroll et al, 1981). Many researchers feel that an abnormal DST is helpful in establishing the diagnosis of a major depressive disorder. It is of the utmost importance, however, to keep in mind that a normal DST is not helpful in ruling out such a disorder, since only 40% to 50% of depressed patients have an abnormal test result.

The DST can also be useful to the clinician faced with patients with confusing or mixed clinical pictures. For example, Greden and Carroll (1979) report a case of a catatonic woman who had an abnormal DST result. Because of this finding, a diagnosis of primary unipolar depression was entertained, and emergency electroconvulsive therapy was begun. She responded rapidly.

There is some preliminary evidence that in nonsuppressing depressed patients, return of normal DST suppression may be a good predictor of when to stop treatment. It is clear that failure to suppress with dexamethasone eventually reverts to a normal dexamethasone response as depression resolves. Some patients, however, may appear clinically to have recovered from their depression but still have an abnormal DST result. Several authors have studied this interesting population. Goldberg (1980a; 1980b) looked at ten patients who had abnormal DST results when depressed and whose medication was stopped after they had been clinically free of depression for one month. The DST was repeated immediately prior to the discontinuation of drug therapy. Of the five patients who showed a normal posttreatment DST result, none had undergone relapse at seven-month follow-up. On the other hand, all five of the patients who continued to show a failure to suppress plasma cortisol levels with dexamethasone, even though clinically healthy, had significant relapses within two months after medication was stopped. In another study, Greden and colleagues found similar results, with only two of ten posttreatment DST suppressors undergoing relapse at follow-up, compared with all four of the patients with abnormal DST results, who underwent relapse after treatment was discontinued (Greden et al, 1980). These preliminary findings indicate that the DST may be a good predictor of when to stop treatment in those depressed patients who initially have an abnormal DST result. An abnormal DST result in a patient free of symptoms may predict an acute relapse.

The DST and Elderly Patients

To determine the clinical usefulness of the DST in geriatric populations, one must know whether the test result is altered in normal elderly persons. Recently, Tourigny-Rivard et al (1981) compared ten healthy elderly (mean age, 75.3) and ten healthy young male (mean age, 29.9) subjects and concluded that advanced age alone did not affect the overnight DST result in healthy subjects and should not invalidate its use as a laboratory tool in the diagnosis and investigation of depression.

One of the common clinical dilemmas facing the physician treating elderly patients is to separate the truly demented patient from the patient who has reversible cognitive impairment on the basis of depression (pseudodementia) (Wells, 1979). If the DST result could be shown to be normal in dementia and abnormal in depression, this would be a great aid to the clinician faced with this dilemma. Unfortunately, there are at present little data, and no firm conclusions can be drawn. A few case reports, however, suggest that the DST may be useful in some instances. Rudorfer and Clayton (1981) reported a patient with pseudodementia whose abnormal DST result normalized after treatment of the underlying depressive illness. Also, Greden and Carroll's (1979) patient originally received the diagnosis of dementia but was later thought to have depression-induced catatonia. Her initially abnormal DST result returned to normal following two courses of electroconvulsive therapy. Similarly, McAllister et al (1982) described two patients for whom the DST appeared to be useful in distinguishing depression with associated severe cognitive deficits from dementia. These reports are encouraging. On the other hand, Spar and Gerner (1982) found abnormal DST results in nine of 17 elderly patients with dementia who did not appear to have major depressive illness. Also, Raskind et al (1982) found that seven of 15 patients with advanced primary degenerative dementia had abnormal DSTs. Clearly, these reports dampen enthusiasm for using the DST to differentiate dementia from pseudodementia, but a few points must be kept in mind when one reviews their findings. First, these patients were severely demented. Spar and Gerner's patients had a mean score of 13.3 out of a possible 30 on the Mini-Mental State Exam and an average duration of symptoms of 4.3 years. The patients of Raskind et al were even further advanced. They had a mean duration of illness of 7.4 years and had no correct responses on the Short Portable Mental Status Questionnaire. In addition, each patient had dysphasia severe enough to grossly impair meaningful speech.

It is well documented that dementia is a multisystem illness, and it is not surprising that neuroendocrine abnormalities exist in patients with advanced disease (see chapter 6). Most patients, however, in whom the diagnostic confusion between depression and dementia occur are only mildly demented. Also, it is impossible to say for certain that the patients with abnormal DST results were not depressed without therapeutic trials of electroconvulsive therapy or pharmacotherapy having been made. Recently, Jenike and Albert (1984) performed the dexamethasone suppression test on 18 patients with presenile and senile dementia of the Alzheimer's type. Objective cognitive testing showed that 13 patients were mild to moderately impaired and five were moderate to severely impaired. The patients were nondepressed on the Hamilton Depression Scale score and also by clinical interview. The DST was abnormal in only one of the mildly impaired patients, but in four of the five moderately impaired patients. These data suggest that the DST may be a useful clinical tool in mildly impaired Alzheimer's patients but is likely to be confounded by disease in moderate to severely impaired patients. These data are consistent with the hypothesis that the DST is not invalidated by *early* Alzheimer's disease.

In summary, the DST is a potentially useful test to aid the clinician in the diagnosis, treatment and follow-up of those elderly patients with suspected depressive illness. In the absence of either medical illness or medication that affects the DST, resistance to dexamethasone suppression strongly suggests the presence of a major depressive disorder. A normal DST does not, however, rule out such a disorder. As more research is done on the DST, it may turn out that the DST is not as specific as it was thought to be initially. It may be a less specific indicator of psychiatric disease, similar to the ESR for inflammatory disorders, of value in screening for psychiatric illness, and in following the course, treatment, and resolution of such disease. Normalization of a previously abnormal DST may be a better guide than the clinical picture to the discontinuation of treatment with antidepressants. Patients who appear to improve clinically but whose DST is still abnormal are at high risk of experiencing significant relapse if treatment is discontinued. When, in the face of an apparent clinical recovery, the DST fails to become normal, the prognosis is poor and the abnormal DST signals the need for continued antidepressant therapy. In nondemented elderly patients, the DST can be used in a manner similar to that used in middle-aged adults. The use of the DST as an aid in the diagnosis of depression in patients with severe dementia is unclear at this time, since some data indicate that dementia alone may produce abnormal DST results. Preliminary data, however, indicate that mild to moderate dementia may not invalidate the DST as a clinical aid in detecting depression.

DRUG TREATMENT OF DEPRESSION

Tricyclic and Heterocyclic Agents

Therapeutic strategy of depression begins with a choice of antidepressant medication, a decision based upon previous treatment response and anticipation of which side effects may pose the greatest problems or produce therapeutic benefits for the patient. Since the introduction of imipramine about 30 years ago, tricyclics have been the mainstay of pharmacologic treatment for depression. As with the neuroleptics, since these agents are generally considered to be equally effective, the choice of drug should be based on side effects. Tertiary amines such as amitriptyline, imipramine, and doxepin are much more likely to cause hypotension than secondary amines such as desipramine, protriptyline, and nortriptyline (Figure 4-3, Table 4-2) (Salzman, 1982). In addition, tertiary amines tend to produce more sedation, presumably by blocking synaptic serotonin reuptake or by affecting histamine receptors (Richelson, 1982).

Anticholinergic and noradrenergic side effects are also particularly troublesome in the elderly (see chapter 8). Anticholinergic symptoms may be prominent both centrally (delirium, confusion, cognitive impairment) and peripherally (tachycardia, urinary retention, constipation, blurred vision, dry mouth, and exacerbation of narrow angle

Table 4-2
Characteristics of Tricyclic and Heterocyclic Agents in Treatment of Depression

Generic Name	Trade Name	Relative Anticholinergic Effect	Sedative Effect	Inhibition of Reuptake	
				Norepinephrine	Serotonin
Tricyclic Tertiary Amines					
Amitriptyline	Elavil and others	8	High	0	4+
Imipramine	Tofranil and others	2	Moderate	2+	3+
Doxepin	Sinequan, Adapin	2	High	0	4+
Tricyclic Secondary Amines					
Desipramine	Norpramin, Pertofrane	1	Low	4+	0
Protriptyline	Vivactil, Triptil	?High	Low	Uncertain	Uncertain
Nortriptyline	Aventyl, Pamelor	2	Moderate	2+	2+
Others					
Amoxapine	Ascendin	2	Moderate	4+	1+
Maprotiline	Ludiomil	2	Moderate	4+	0
Trazodone	Desyrel	0	High	0	4+

Reproduced with permission from Jenike MA: Drug treatment of depression. *Topics in Geriatrics* 2:10, 1983.

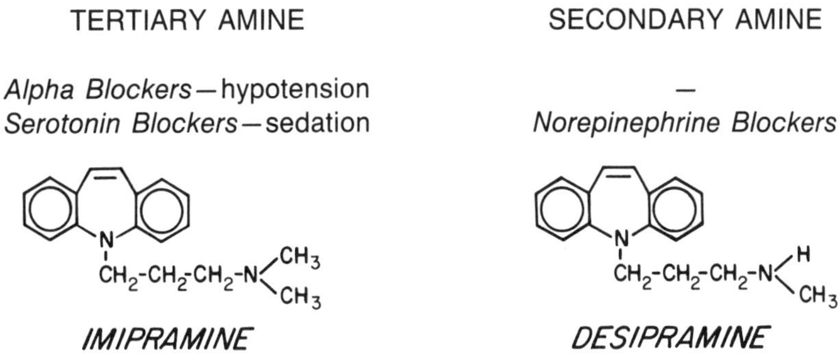

TERTIARY AMINE	SECONDARY AMINE
Alpha Blockers—hypotension Serotonin Blockers—sedation	— Norepinephrine Blockers

IMIPRAMINE   DESIPRAMINE

Figure 4-3   Tertiary vs. secondary amines.

glaucoma). If desipramine (Norpramin) is assigned an anticholinergic potency of 1, amitriptyline (Elavil) would be eight times more anticholinergic. The other tricyclics lie somewhere in between with a relative potency of about 2 (Table 4-2). There is also some recent data that suggests that protriptyline (Vivactil) may be the worse offender among the tricyclics for atropinelike side effects (Cassem, 1982; Tollefson et al, 1982). Clinically, however, amitriptyline is generally regarded as the tricyclic most likely to cause a clinically hazardous tachycardia (Cassem, 1982). The combination of pronounced anticholinergic activity and danger of orthostatic hypotension makes amitriptyline the least desirable of all the available tricyclics used to treat depression (Jenike, 1983a). Based on in vitro comparisons of anticholinergic potency, one might estimate that amitriptyline is about one-twentieth as active as atropine at central and peripheral muscarinic cholinergic receptors, so that a daily dose of 150 mg of amitriptyline corresponds to approximately 7.5 mg of atropine, a dose which would almost never be given (Cassem, 1982).

If a patient has had a prior positive response or if he has a relative who had a good outcome from a particular drug, it may be best to begin treatment with this drug. In general, tertiary amine tricyclics and agents with high anticholinergic potency should be avoided in the elderly. The choice of antidepressant can be based largely on the clinical picture. For instance, if a depressed patient is sleeping much more than usual and requires an activating (noradrenergic) agent, desipramine (Norpramin) would be a good drug to try. If, on the other hand, the patient is unable to sleep, more sedating agents like nortriptyline (Aventyl, Pamelor), trazodone (Desyrel), or maprotiline (Ludiomil) should be started.

Amoxapine (Ascendin), first available in the United States in 1981, is the demethylated derivative of the antipsychotic loxapine and is comparable in efficacy to the standard tricyclic agents (Dominquez, 1983). Hypotension is an uncommon side effect, but several cases of seizures have been reported. Amoxapine inhibits both norepinephrine and serotonin reuptake, and also blocks dopamine receptors and produces extrapyramidal side effects typical of neuroleptics. It has been reported to cause acute dystonia, parkinsonism, and akathisia (Lydiard and Gelenberg, 1981; Barton, 1982; Jenike, 1983e), and there is a recent report of tardive dyskinesia associated with amoxapine use (Lapierre and Anderson, 1983). Since the elderly are particularly prone to develop tardive dyskinesia, and since the movements associated with it are much less likely to be reversible in older individuals (Jenike, 1983d), amoxapine should be avoided in elderly patients suffering from uncomplicated depression. In patients who are both psychotic and depressed, amoxapine may be a reasonable drug to use for short periods of time (Jenike, 1983e).

Maprotiline (Ludiomil), also introduced in 1981, is a tetracyclic that is very similar to standard tricyclics in its action (Dominquez, 1983). It is a specific blocker of norepinephrine reuptake, with apparently no effect on serotonin uptake. It has little anticholinergic effect and does not commonly produce orthostatic hypotension. In addition, it appears to have a lower incidence of cardiovascular side effects (Wells and Gelenberg, 1981). Seizures have been reported and skin rashes occur in up to 10% of patients (Dominquez, 1983).

In early 1982, trazodone (Desyrel) was introduced into the United States. It has a different structure than other antidepressant agents and is a selective, serotonin uptake blocker. It is similar in efficacy to the standard tricyclics (Murphy and Ankier, 1980), but has a very low incidence of anticholinergic side effects, although clinically some patients complain of dry mouth. The lack of anticholinergic side effects with trazodone is probably responsible for the low incidence of therapy dropouts in comparative studies with tricyclics and other agents (Newton, 1981). The elderly seem to tolerate trazodone very well. Clinically, trazodone is sedating and is particularly helpful for depressed patients who cannot sleep. Other common side effects include indigestion, nausea, and headaches. Trazodone appears to have a more benign cardiac side effect profile compared with the tricyclics (Himmelhoch, 1981). Caution is still recommended in using trazodone in patients with preexisting cardiac disease. It appears to be particularly nonmalignant when taken in overdose; at this point, there have been no life-threatening complications after trazodone overdose such as those frequently associated with overdose of tricyclic antidepressants.

It is important to remember that the dosing schedule is different from most of the other agents we use. Roughly 400 mg of trazodone is equivalent to 150 mg of amitriptyline or imipramine. Clinicians frequently underdose patients with trazodone.

Because of its presumed lack of side effects, trazodone appears particularly suited for use in elderly patients. Since digoxin is frequently prescribed in this population, a possible interaction between trazodone and digoxin should be kept in mind. The following case was recently reported (Rauch and Jenike, 1984) and is reproduced here with permission:

> *Case:* A 68-year-old woman with a 30-year history of unipolar affective illness was admitted to our inpatient psychiatry service for treatment of severe depression of three weeks' duration. The symptoms, which were characteristic of past depressions, included loss of appetite, lack of energy, disinterest in her appearance, severe anxiety, and refusal to get out of bed. The medical history was significant for congestive heart failure, hypertension, atrial tachyarrhythmia, and impaired renal function presumed secondary to hypertensive nephropathy. Previously, she had undergone a modified radical mastectomy for cancer in the left breast with one positive lymph node and no further evidence of metastatic disease.
>
> On admission, she was medically stable and was receiving digoxin, clonidine, quinidine gluconate, and a triamterene-hydrochlorothiazide combination. The digoxin levels had remained within therapeutic ranges for many months on the same dosage (125 μg/day of digoxin), as did the quinidine levels. The results of laboratory tests on admission were within normal limits except for a slightly elevated creatinine value of 1.3 mg/100 mL with a BUN of 24 mg/100 mL. The admission digoxin level was 0.8 ng/mL (therapeutic range 1.2 to 1.7 ng/mL) and the quinidine level was 4.0 μg/mL (therapeutic range 1.5 to 5.0 μg/mL).
>
> Trazodone 50 mg at bedtime was begun (Day 1 of therapy). It was increased by 50 mg every other day until a dose of 300 mg/d was reached (Day 11). On Day 12 she felt less anxious and the staff reported that she was more sociable and attentive to self-care. On Day 14 she complained of nausea and vomiting. The digoxin level was measured in the toxic range at 2.8 ng/mL while the quinidine level was within therapeutic limits at 1.6 μg/mL. Digoxin was temporarily discontinued and the nausea and vomiting resolved over the next three days. On Day 19 of therapy she had a further elevated creatinine value of 1.9 mg/100 mL with a BUN of 30 mg/100 mL, which returned to baseline levels after fluid intake was increased.
>
> She continued on trazodone, 100 mg in the morning and 200 mg at bedtime. After the digoxin level returned to the therapeutic range, she was switched to 125 μg every other day, which produced therapeutic levels. She continues to be free of her depressive symptoms.

This patient not only developed toxic digoxin levels after starting trazodone, but also required only half her previous maintenance dose of digoxin. This case is complicated by the presence of compromised renal function. There was, however, no change in renal function to account for the lowered maintenance dose of digoxin after trazodone was begun. In a canine model, Dec et al found no elevation in serum digoxin concentration when trazodone was administered with digoxin (Dec et al, 1984). The authors noted that the inability to reproduce a trazodone-digoxin interaction could be due to differences in canine metabolism and excretion of digoxin or trazodone. Canine elimination of digoxin is predominantly renal and more rapid than that observed in humans. Until more data are available, trazodone should be used cautiously in combination with digoxin. In particular, digoxin levels should be closely monitored when trazodone is used concomitantly.

Prior to starting any antidepressant medication, an ECG should be performed on all elderly patients. Treatment should begin with a very low dose—a maximum of 25 mg for most patients (except 5 mg for protriptyline and 50 mg for trazodone). The dosage can be raised slowly every few days. Subjective response and heart rate must be monitored and the clinician must be on the alert for anticholinergic, cardiovascular, or CNS side effects. Dosage increase should be slowed if tachycardia, excessive sedation, or orthostatic hypotension develop. Often the patient is the last to know that he is getting better and family members commonly report that the patient is sleeping and eating better before the dysphoria resolves. An adequate trial takes at least four weeks and probably six weeks at therapeutic levels. Theoretically, drug trials should include at least one noradreneric drug and one serotonergic drug (Table 4-2) (Maas, 1975). Drugs should not be changed, however, until an adequate therapeutic trial is completed; Quitkin and coworkers reviewed drug trials involving patients on a representative spectrum of antidepressants, and found that 40% of patients unresponsive at four weeks responded to treatment if the drug trial was extended to six weeks (Quitkin et al, 1984).

Table 4-3
Suggested Blood Levels for Some Tricyclic Agents (Task Force)

Drug	What Is Measured	Total Therapeutic Level
Imipramine	Imipramine and desipramine	> 200 ng/mL
Desipramine	Desipramine	> 125 ng/mL
Amitriptyline	Amitriptyline and nortriptyline	> 160 ng/mL†
Nortriptyline	Nortriptyline	50–150 ng/mL*
Doxepin	Doxepin and desmethyldoxepin	> 100 ng/mL†

*Therapeutic window: above or below these levels is associated with decreased response.
†Rough estimates.

If these agents are not helpful after a reasonable trial, a blood level determination (when available) will assist the clinician in determining the next step (Table 4-3). They should be drawn in the morning *before* the morning dose of medication. With the same dose, blood levels can vary from ten to as much as 30 times among individuals. Nortriptyline appears to be unique among these agents in that it has a therapeutic window; that is, levels above as well as below the therapeutic range are associated with a decreased response. When the level is not in the appropriate range, dosage should be adjusted.

Heterocyclic Antidepressant Overdose (Gelenberg, 1984)

Each year in the United States, 5000 to 10,000 patients try to poison themselves with antidepressants and about 0.7% of these die (Moriarty, 1981). A recent study reviewed the records of 47 patients who had overdosed on antidepressants (Nicotra et al, 1981) and found that amitriptyline (Elavil) and doxepin (Adapin, Sinequan) were taken most often. Of the 47 patients, three died: one with cardiopulmonary arrest on admission, the other two with respiratory failure after prolonged courses. Half of the patients required respiratory support, usually for less than 48 hours. Seizures that occurred in the course of hospitalization were all grand mal and abated without treatment. A number of cardiovascular effects were reported. Two patients had cardiac arrests prior to admission but were successfully resuscitated. Tachycardia was common on admission, but usually cleared within a day. Hypotension occurred in over a quarter of the cases. Electrocardiographic changes included premature atrial and ventricular contractions as well as prolongation of the PR and QTc intervals.

The relationship between plasma antidepressant levels and clinical evidence of toxicity was unclear. For example, although it has been said that patients with plasma antidepressant levels in excess of 1000 ng/mL usually have QRS complexes greater than 100 ms, Nicotra and colleagues found that this was not always the case; one patient with a level of 3340 ng/mL had a normal QRS complex. In addition, patients with only modestly elevated plasma levels upon hospital admission were not necessarily safe from cardiovascular toxicity. Nicotra et al believed that monitoring the plasma concentration of antidepressants in overdose cases is of limited value and can be misleading. Because the drugs are highly lipophilic and also bind extensively to protein and tissue, plasma levels may reflect only a small portion of the drug available to brain, heart, and other organs. In addition, different organs in different patients may develop tolerance at different rates.

Pentel and Sioris (1981) attempted to determine how frequently unexpected life-threatening arrhythmias occur after antidepressant overdose. Dangerous cardiac events have been reported as long as six days after ingestion. This has a bearing on the question of how long patients who take overdoses should undergo cardiac monitoring. To address this question, they reviewed the charts of all adults hospitalized at a medical center over a four-year period after tricyclic antidepressant overdoses. Amitriptyine, imipramine, and doxepin were the most commonly ingested tricyclic agents in the 129 patients reviewed. Ninety-six of the patients had also taken some other drug at the same time. Mortality in their series was 5.4% (seven patients), five due to ventricular arrhythmias. Four died within one hour of arrival at the hospital, two were pronounced brain dead several days later following intractable arrhythmias and hypotension, and the seventh patient died of pulmonary emboli 24 hours after ingesting a relatively small amount of antidepressant. *All patients who developed arrhythmias or conduction delays on the ECG showed these abnormalities within one hour of hospitalization. Furthermore, once a presenting ECG abnormality had resolved, no patient experienced further cardiac difficulties. No patient developed an arrhythmia after being alert and having a normal ECG for one hour.*

Pentel and Sioris noted that in the previously reported cases of arrhythmias or sudden deaths occurring as long as six days after an antidepressant overdose, patients were never free from CNS or cardiac toxicity prior to the event. Rather, their courses were characterized by major complications such as severe ECG abnormalities, hypotension, and coma. The authors conclude that whereas arrhythmias and death can follow antidepressant ingestion by a number of days, life-threatening events appear to result from serious ongoing complications of the overdose, rather than appearing unexpectedly after a benign interval. On the basis of their review, the authors recommend the following: *After an antidepressant overdose, if (1) a patient is clinically normal, and (2) the EKG is stable for 24 hours, and (3) no contra-active or supportive therapy is required, and (4) the patient does not have a pre-existing cardiac problem, then intensive monitoring may be discontinued.*

In a comprehensive review of the treatment of tricyclic antidepressant overdoses, Jackson and Bressler (1982) have highlighted a number of important aspects of diagnosis and management. For one, they emphasize the importance of other drugs that might be ingested along with the antidepressant. These other drugs, as well as ancillary medical problems, can complicate a clinical picture. For example, seizures that follow a tricyclic overdose could be attributed to the antidepressant, yet they may reflect hypoxia or hypoglycemia. Therefore, the authors recommend the IV administration of naloxone (Narcan) and glucose to patients with seizures and, for that matter, to all comatose or obtunded patients — in case opiates or hypoglycemia may be present.

Similar to the findings of the Nicotra group, Jackson and Bressler report the most common cardiovascular findings in tricyclic overdose cases as sinus tachycardia, hypotension, prolonged QRS complexes, and prolonged PR and OT intervals. Less frequent, but more ominous, are other supraventricular tachycardias, intraventricular conduction defects, atrioventricular (AV) block, bradycardia, nodal rhythms, and ventricular irritability.

As a general therapeutic measure, the authors stress the importance of maintaining adeduate ventilation — via mechanical means, if necessary. Once vital functions are stabilized, any unabsorbed drug should be removed from the gastrointestinal (GI) tract. Because of their anticholinergic activity, antidepressants (and other psychotropic compounds) may be present in the stomach for many hours after an overdose. Ipecac, which can be of some use at home immediately after ingestion, should not be administered in the face of ileus or to a stuporous or unresponsive patient. Rather, gastric lavage should be performed with a large (34 F or larger) orogastric tube. (Small nasogastric tubes cannot remove concretions of tablets.) Administration of a cathartic, such as castor oil, and activated charcoal, 50 to 100 g should follow. Because of enterohepatic recirculation of active antidepressant metabolites, castor oil and charcoal should be repeated every eight to 12 hours. The authors note that late-occurring toxicity following an overdose could be related to delayed absorption of drugs that have remained in the GI tract — which underscores the importance of prompt and complete removal.

When seizures occur following an antidepressant overdose, physostigmine (Antilirium) may be administered. However, the authors are extremely wary of this approach, noting the paradoxical possibility of increased seizures, as well as enhanced overall mortality. Among standard anticonvulsants, diazepam (Valium) is probably the most effective; phenytoin (Dilantin and others) seems relatively ineffective in these circumstances.

Recently four cases of overdose with amoxapine (Ascendin) were reported where all patients developed severe, multiple seizures. Physostigmine, 2 to 8 mg, was ineffective in treating the seizures. In one particularly severe case, seizures were similarly refractory to treatment with diazepam, 300 mg, and thiopental sodium (Pentothal) 1200 mg (Krenzelok and North, 1981). Goldberg and Spector (1982) reported two cases of amoxapine overdose, which resulted in severe and persistent impairment of the CNS. The first was that of a 24-year-old, previously healthy woman, who took approximately 4 g of amoxapine. (The maximum dose recommended by the manufacturer is 600 mg daily in divided doses.) At the hospital, she was treated with gastric lavage, then activated charcoal and a saline cathartic and, because of an elevated body temperature, a cooling blanket. Soon after, she had a tonic-clonic seizure, followed by severe metabolic acidosis and hypokalemia. The patient developed recurrent seizures and fell into a deep coma, requiring endotracheal intubation and mechanical ventilation. Seizures persisted for about eight hours and were refractory through IV phenytoin, diazepam, phenobarbital, and physostigmine. However, she never became hypotensive, hypertensive, hypoxemic, or oliguric, and her vital signs, blood gases, and urine output remained stable. Her neurologic condition improved gradually over seven months, but at three months after the overdose she could speak only in short phases with dysarthria, had severe memory deficits and poor judgment, and required ongoing nursing care. They saw an almost identical case of a 29-year-old woman who had taken at least 2 g of amoxapine, and who also developed multiple seizures and severe metabolic acidosis and remained comatose for two weeks. Four weeks after her overdose, this patient too was still hospitalized with neurologic symptoms similar to the preceding woman's.

Kulig and collaborators (Kulig et al, 1982) have described an additional five cases of amoxapine overdoses, noting seizures in each, but relatively benign cardiovascular effects. The wide age range included a 6-year-old boy, a 51-year-old woman, and two women and a man in their 30s. Each of these patients went through a period of coma, and two required endotracheal intubation. All patients recovered fully, although the course of one patient was complicated by rhabdomyolysis, myoglobinuria, and renal failure. In particular, cardiovascular reactions to the overdose were surprisingly mild, — little more than sinus tachycardia — which the authors contrast with the complications often observed with tricyclic antidepressant overdoses. The possibility that amoxapine overdose may cause a greater incidence of seizures, but a lower incidence of cardiotoxicity, is worth considering, although it remains unproven.

The most recent report on amoxapine toxicity is by Litovitz and Trautman (1983), who reviewed all ingestions reported to poison centers in Washington, DC and New Mexico over an 18-month period between 1980 and 1982. Of all reported overdoses, 479 included heterocyclic antidepressants, 33 of which were amoxapine. Fifteen of the amoxapine overdose patients developed "substantial toxic conditions." Eight (24%) became comatose. Thirteen (9%) had supraventricular tachycardia. Twelve (36%) suffered seizures. Hyperthermia developed in three patients (9%), all of whom sustained prolonged convulsions. Two patients (6%) developed a coagulopathy, and one of these had profuse hemorrhage. *Five patients (15.2%) died.* By contrast, of 446 patients who took excessive amounts of other antidepressants, 19 (4%) had seizures and three (less than 1%) died. Previous reports had noted the high frequency of seizures in amoxapine overdoses; the general impression, however, had been that amoxapine was less likely than other heterocyclic compounds to produce fatalities. Against this background, Litovitz and Trautman's report is most worrisome. Cases reported to regional poison centers are not all inclusive and are therefore open to possible bias; however, the number of cases reported by these authors is impressive and substantially extends the data base on amoxapine overdoses. Appropriate caution should be exercised in prescribing any antidepressant to patients with a seizure diathesis, but confirming whether some of the newer antidepressants may be more hazardous in this regard must await additional information.

Overdose-induced cardiac arrhythmias often respond well to alkalinization with IV sodium bicarbonate, may respond to phenytoin, and might possibly be decreased with β-blockers (eg, propranolol [Inderal]). It is important to avoid type I antiarrhythmics — quinidine, procainamide hydrochloride (Pronestyl), and disopyramide phosphate (Norpace) — which tend to aggravate the effects of a tricyclic on the cardiac conduction system and myocardium.

If antidepressant-induced impairment of cardiac rhythm results in diminished (or absent) hemoperfusion, external support of ventilation and cardiac output (ie, cardiopulmonary resuscitation) should be continued for a longer period — hours, if necessary. In previously healthy patients, this support can allow metabolism and distribution of the offending agent, with the possibility of full recovery (Orr and Bramble, 1981).

As new antidepressant agents become available, the problem of serious toxicity from overdoses may diminish. For example, trazodone (Desyrel) is said to be much less toxic when taken in excess. At this point there are no reported fatalities when trazodone has been taken alone in overdose. But while the more toxic antidepressants remain with us, so will the risk of overdose. And for that reason, physicians should be careful to assess the suicide potential of patients to whom they prescribe these drugs. Furthermore, patients should be seen frequently during the early days of therapy, both to increase clinical monitoring and to diminish the amount of antidepressants that must be prescribed at each visit. Since elderly patients are at high risk for suicide and are particularly vulnerable to the malignant side effects of these agents when taken in overdose, these issues are of the utmost importance.

Monoamine Oxidase Inhibitors (MAOIs)

Among the somatic treatments available for treating depressed patients, the MAOIs are the least used. Many clinicians avoid the use of MAOIs in elderly patients because of fears of adverse reactions. In fact, many textbooks of geriatrics make no mention of the use of MAOIs for the elderly. It is now known that these agents can be safely used for the elderly when certain precautions are taken. Many patients who do not respond to tricyclics or some of the newer antidepressants will improve with MAOIs. Also, MAOIs have been found to be especially effective in treating depression related to dementia (Ashford and Ford, 1979; Jenike, 1985). The following is an example of a not uncommon case (Jenike, 1984b).

> *Case*: Mr. A, a 72-year-old retired laborer, was brought to the psychiatric memory disorders clinic of Massachusetts General Hospital with a one-year history of worsening memory. In addition, the patient's wife told us that he had become increasingly withdrawn and was losing interest in his hobbies. Previously an avid traveler, he now wanted to just sit at home, often alone and in the dark. He was refusing to drive, had lost his appetite, with a resultant weight loss of 12 pounds, and seemed frequently confused and unable to concentrate. He denied any suicidal ideation but admitted to feeling very depressed and hopeless. He had a strong family history of depression and his mother had received electroconvulsive therapy on one occasion, with good result.
>
> Results from Mr. A's dementia workup were entirely negative, and neuropsychiatric testing results were consistent with the initial impression that Mr. A was suffering from an affective illness with secondary memory impairment (pseudodementia).
>
> Mr. A was started on desipramine, 25 mg at bedtime, and the dose was increased slowly to 200 mg daily. He suffered no side effects but also got no better over the next eight weeks, despite measured blood levels in the therapeutic range. Desipramine eventually discontinued and nortriptyline was begun, starting with a low dosage. Once again he failed to respond despite blood levels in therapeutic range.
>
> Because Mr. A had not improved on two tricyclic antidepressants and the family feared electroconvulsive therapy, a MAOI was begun. After a ten-day drug-free period, tranylcypromine was started at 10 mg twice a day and slowly increased to 20 mg twice a day. After two weeks, Mr. A was much improved, and within eight weeks he was

"back to his former self." He has continued on tranylcypromine and, at a return visit to the clinic three months later, was observed to be doing well. Repeat clinical testing at that time showed that his cognitive disturbances had resolved.

Precautions and side effects of MAOIs   It is essential that all patients on MAOIs receive dietary and drug precautions (Tables 4-4 and 4-5) (Sheehan et al, 1980-1981; Jenike, 1984b). Elderly patients comply well and rarely complain about such restrictions. A low tyramine diet is required, necessitating avoidance of foods such as fermented cheese, yogurt, beer, red wine, and excessive amounts of caffeine and chocolate. Patients can safely drink white wine, vodka, gin, and whiskey, and a blanket instruction to avoid all alcohol is not only unwarranted but also may decrease compliance dramatically (Jenike, 1983f). Combination cold tablets, nasal decongestants, appetite suppressors, and amphetamines must be avoided. Pure antihistamines, such as chlorpheniramine, however, can safely be used to treat patients who have rhinitis (Table 4-4) (Jenike, 1983f; 1984b).

There is a poorly understood toxic interaction between MAOIs and meperidine hydrochloride, which was first described in 1955 (Mitchell, 1955) and has been reported occasionally since that time (Meyer and Halfin, 1981). Clinically, patients appear agitated, disoriented, cyanotic, hyperthermic, hypertensive, and tachycardic. This toxic interaction can be fatal. Should this occur, chlorpromazine has been used as an effective treatment (Papp and Benaim, 1958; Jenike, 1984b). There have been no clinical reports of the same severe toxic interactions with other narcotics, although increased potency has been noted experimentally in animals (Meyer and Halfin, 1981). Should narcotics be needed for a patient on a MAOI, a prudent course would be to begin with half the usual dosage and titrate the dosage slowly on the basis of symptomatic response, bearing in mind that increased potency will be more pronounced if the narcotic is given close to the time that the MAOI was taken that day (Meyer and Halfin, 1981).

Because MAOIs have essentially no anticholinergic effects, they are useful for patients who are sensitive to these side effects. For example, the elderly patient who has urinary retention with only a 10-mg dosage of dcsipramine hydrochloride may do very well on a MAOI. MAOIs generally are more stimulating and less sedating than tricyclic antidepressants. Some women taking MAOIs are unable to achieve orgasm (*The Medical Letter,* July 11, 1980, p 58). Serious hepatic toxicity, which used to occur frequently with earlier MAOIs, is rare with those currently available.

Table 4-4
Dietary Restrictions for Patients Taking Monoamine Oxidase Inhibitors

---

	FOODS
***	All cheese
***	All foods containing cheese, eg, pizza, fondue, many Italian dishes, salad dressings
Safe	Fresh cottage cheese, cream cheese, yogurt in moderate amounts
**	Sour cream
**	All fermented or aged foods, especially aged meats or aged fish, eg, aged corned beef, salami, fermented sausage (pepperoni, summer sausage), pickled herring
**	Liver (chicken, beef, or pork liver)
**	Liverwurst
***	Broad bean *pods* (English bean pods, Chinese pea pods)
**	Meat extracts or yeast extracts, eg, Bovril or Marmite
Safe	Baked products raised with yeast, eg, bread
Safe	Yeast
**	Spoiled or dried fruit, eg, spoiled bananas, figs, raisins
Safe	Fresh fruits, except pineapple and avocados

The following foods have been rarely reported to cause hypertensive reactions with MAOIs. The evidence supporting these claims is weak and often based on a single isolated case. Warnings based on such evidence have been uncritically perpetuated, especially in view of the large numbers of patients on MAOIs who have eaten these foods with no problem. In practice a blanket prohibition of these foods seems unjustified, unless they are clearly spoiled or decayed, except for specific patients in whom they have already caused symptoms.

*	Chocolate
*	Anchovies
*	Caviar
*	Coffee
*	Colas
*	Sauerkraut
*	Mushrooms
*	Beet root (beets)
*	Rhubarb
*	Curry powder
*	Junket
*	Worcestershire sauce
*	Soy sauce
*	Licorice
*	Snails

	DRINKS
**	Red wine, sherry, vermouth, cognac
**	Beer and ale
Safe	Other alcoholic drinks, eg, gin, vodka, whiskey, in true moderation

Table 4-4 (continued)

	DRUGS
***	Cold medications, eg, Dristan, Contact
***	Nasal decongestants, sinus medicine
***	Asthma inhalants
Safe	Pure steroid asthma inhalants, eg, beclomethasone dipropionate (Vanceril)
**	Allergy and hay fever medications
Safe	Pure antihistamines (chlorpheniramine, brompheniramine)
***	Meperidine (Demerol)
Safe	Other narcotics (eg, codeine) in lowered doses
***	Amphetamines
**	Antiappetite (diet) medicine
	Sympathomimetic amines
**	Direct-acting: eg, epinephrine, isoproterenol, methoxamine, norepinephrine
***	Indirect-acting: eg, amphetamines, methylphenidate, phenylpropanolamine, ephedrine, cyclopentamine, pseudoephedrine, tyramine
***	Direct- and indirect-acting: eg, metaraminol, phenylephrine
**	Local anesthetics with epinephrine
Safe	Local anesthetics without epinephrine, eg, mepivacaine (Carbocaine)
**	Levodopa for parkinsonism
**	Dopamine
Safe	Diabetics on insulin may have increased hypoglycemia requiring a decreased dose of insulin, but insulin is otherwise safe
Safe	Patients on hypotensive agents for high blood pressure may have more hypotension, requiring a decrease in their use of hypotensive agent, which otherwise is safe

Danger of Rise in Blood Pressure: *Minimal danger, **Moderate danger, ***Very dangerous.
Reproduced with permission from Jenike MA: The use of monoamine oxidase inhibitors in the treatment of elderly, depressed patients. *J Am Geriatr Soc* 32:571-575, 1984.

The side effects of MAOIs that cause the most problems for the elderly are hypotension and insomnia. Insomnia can be minimized by giving the last daily dose no later than 4 PM. Some patients, however, feel drowsy on these agents, particularly phenelzine sulfate, and can be given the drug at bedtime. It is best to start with a daytime dosing schedule and switch to evenings only if the patient complains of drowsiness. Orthostatic hypotension is the more dangerous side effect for geriatric patients, because they tolerate falls poorly. It had been thought that MAOI-induced orthostatic hypotension occurred early in the course of treatment and that if patients could tolerate the first few days of medication, hypotension would rarely necessitate discontinuing the drug (Mielke, 1976: Robinson et al, 1978; Jenike 1983g). Recently, however, Kronig and associates (1983) carefully followed a small group of patients (n = 14; average age 52) and reported that the mean orthostatic

Table 4-5
Instructions for Patients Taking Monoamine Oxidase Inhibitors

Avoid all the food and drugs mentioned on the dietary restrictions list. Be particularly careful to avoid those foods and drugs with two and three stars.

In general, all of the foods you should avoid are decayed, fermented, or aged in some way. Avoid any aged food even if it is not on the list.

If you get a cold or flu, you may use aspirin, or Tylenol. For a cough, glycerin cough drops or plain Robitussin may be used.

All laxatives or stool softeners may be used for constipation.

All antibiotics, eg, penicillin, tetracycline, and erythromycin, may be safely used to treat infections.

Avoid all other medications without first checking with me. This includes any over-the-counter medicines bought without prescription, eg, cold tablets, nose drops, cough medicine, diet pills.

Eating one of the restricted foods may cause a sudden elevation of your blood pressure. When this occurs, you get an explosive headache, particularly in the back of your head and temples. Your head and face will feel flushed and full, your heart may pound, and you may perspire heavily and feel nauseated.

If you need medical or dental care while on this medication, show these restrictions and instructions to the doctor. Have the doctor call my office _____ if they have any questions or need further clarification or information.

Side effects such as postural lightheadedness, constipation, delay in urination, delay in ejaculation and orgasm, muscle twitching, sedation, fluid retention, insomnia, and excess sweating are quite common. Many of these side effects lessen considerably after the third week.

Lightheadedness may occur following sudden changes in position. This can be avoided by getting up slowly. If tablets are taken with meals, this and the other side effects are lessened.

The medication is rarely effective in less than three weeks.

Care should be taken while operating any machinery or while driving, since some patients have episodes of sleepiness in the early phases of treatment with MAO inhibitors.

Take the medication precisely as directed. Do not regulate the number of pills without first consulting me.

In spite of the side effects and special dietary restrictions, your medication, an MAO inhibitor, is safe and effective when take as directed.

If any special problems arise, call me at my office.

See also Table 4-4.
Reproduced with permission from Jenike MA: The use of monoamine oxidase inhibitors in the treatment of elderly, depressed patients. *J Am Geriatr Soc* 32:571–575, 1984.

drop increased with time and peaked between three and four weeks after MAOIs were begun. Their data imply that clinicians should continue to watch for orthostatic changes at least throughout the first month of treatment.

The most important adverse effect associated with MAOIs is the uncommon, but frightening, occurrence of a hypertensive crisis caused by a toxic interaction with certain drugs or tyramine-containing foods. Tyramine and other amines can cause hypertension by a mechanism that is not completely understood. Normally, ingested tyramine is inactivated by monoamine oxidase in the GI tract and liver; when this is prevented by MAOIs, palpitations, severe headaches and hypertensive crisis can result (*The Medical Letter,* July 11, 1980, p 58). The elderly patient who has fragile atherosclerotic blood vessels could easily suffer a stroke during such a crisis. Intravenous phentolamine, an α-adrenergic blocker, is recommended for treatment of severe hypertensive reactions. Alternatively, chlorpromazine, which has α-adrenergic blocking activity, can be given IM. One systematic study of dietary noncompliance showed that although nearly 40% of 98 patients taking tranylcypromine sulfate acknowledged "cheating" on their restrictions, no serious complications ensued (Neil et al, 1979).

Little is gained by measuring platelet MAO activity while patients are on these agents. The assay is generally not readily available and some researchers have found no significant relationships between clinical response and platelet MAO inhibition (Davidson and White, 1983). Also, White and colleagues found that MAO inhibition levels were not consistent and could vary with assay methodology, laboratory technique, and gender unmatched comparison groups (White et al, 1983).

At the Massachusetts General Hospital we have for a number of years routinely used MAOIs as maintenance therapy for patients who have received electroconvulsive therapy for severe depressive disorders. Most of these patients are over the age of 60 years. To my knowledge, we have not had a single patient develop a hypertensive episode; the overwhelming majority tolerate these agents very well. Tranylcypromine is our preferred MAOI for elderly patients because it is a reversible enzyme blocker which, when discontinued, will be out of the patient's system within 24 hours. In contra-distinction, phenelzine irreversibly blocks MAO, and its effects may persist for over a week when discontinued (Goodman and Gilman, 1975). Our usual starting dose of tranylcypromine is 10 mg twice daily. Most elderly patients can be treated effectively on this dose, but some may require gradual increase to 60 mg daily. Phenelzine should be started at 15 mg twice daily and may need to be increased slowly to as high as 90 mg for some patients.

There are no known long-term adverse effects of MAOIs, such as the tardive dyskinesia that occurs with chronic use of neuroleptics.

The following conclusions may be drawn with regard to MAOIs:

1. MAOIs are safe and effective for the elderly when certain simple precautions are taken.
2. Give patients a list of foods to avoid (Table 4-4) and an instruction sheet (Table 4-5). Advise them not to take any medications that are not listed as safe on the instruction sheet unless they check with a physician.
3. To lessen chances of insomnia, give the last dose of medication before 4 PM.
4. Reasonable starting doses are 10 mg twice daily for tranylcypromine or 15 mg twice daily for phenelzine. Maintain elderly patients on this dose for at least one week and increase the dose slowly.
5. Monitor blood pressure for orthostatic changes for at least one month, as recent evidence indicates that such changes may not be present initially.
6. If a hypertensive crisis develops, phentolamine or chlorpromazine can be used for rapid blood pressure control.
7. Do not administer meperidine for pain relief to patients taking MAOIs. Other narcotics can be used safely, but should be started at a lower than usual dosage.

Lithium

Lithium is not used frequently in the elderly. It is unusual for mania to occur initially past the age of 65 and most elderly patients who present in a manic state have a history of prior manic episodes (Jefferson, 1983). Only about 5% of patients admitted to psychogeriatric wards suffer from manic episodes. Of those elderly patients admitted for affective disorders, Roth found that 13% were suffering predominantly from manic symptoms (Roth, 1955).

The median age of onset for bipolar illness is 30 years; the risk of illness remains fairly high until age 50 and then decreases sharply. Almost 90% of all cases have onset before age 50 years (Angst et al, 1973). Early-onset bipolar disorder is an illness that usually continues into later life; so even though the initial onset of bipolar disorder may be rare after age 65, the bipolar population that eventually reaches old age will be substantial. The New York State Psychiatric Institute Lithium Clinic reported that about 20% of 200 active patients were over 65 years of age (Dunner et al, 1979).

As in younger patients, the primary uses of lithium in the elderly are to treat mania and prevent recurrent episodes in bipolar patients. Lithium has also been used with some success in schizoaffective disorder and recurrent unipolar depression (Jefferson, 1983). The utility of lithium in treating acute depression is not well established although occasional lithium-responsive bipolar and unipolar depressives are reported (Jefferson, 1983). Lithium is not the drug of first choice for depression in elderly patients, but may be a useful adjuvant in tricyclic antidepressant-resistant unipolar depressed patients. DeMontigny and associates (deMontigny et al, 1981) reported that eight such patients (aged 33 to 64 years) responded within 48 hours when lithium was added to the tricyclic regimen.

Based on little data, it appears that lithium is just as effective in the elderly as it is in younger patients. In patients with coexisting organic brain syndrome, however, lithium is reportedly less effective and is associated with increased risk (Jefferson, 1983).

Special precautions in the elderly   As mentioned in chapter 2, the glomerular filtration rate (GFR) decreases with advancing age (Rowe et al, 1976). Since lithium is almost exclusively excreted by the kidneys, dosage modification will be routinely required and in patients with renal disease, drastic reductions in dose will be needed.

Elderly patients tend to have more diseases than younger patients. These acute and chronic illnesses can complicate lithium use in the elderly. For example, superimposed renal disease not only impairs lithium excretion, but also may increase chances of lithium-induced nephrotoxicity. Dementing illnesses may sensitize a patient to lithium-induced neurotoxicity and also decrease ability to comply with dosing schedules (Himmelhoch et al, 1980). Cardiovascular disease may make patients vulnerable to fluid and electrolyte alterations and may increase risk of cardiotoxicity (Jefferson, 1983).

Elderly patients with more disease will be on multiple medications. Not only will there be an increased incidence of side effects, but it will be harder to establish which drug is responsible for which side effect. Also, compliance problems will increase and there will be an increased likelihood of adverse drug interactions.

Common drug interactions with lithium   Because many elderly patients suffer from idiopathic hypertension, thiazide diuretics are frequently taken in combination with lithium. They consistently cause decreased renal clearance of lithium and raise serum lithium levels. Whenever a thiazide is added to ongoing lithium therapy, dosage will generally have to be lowered. Conversely, to avoid subtherapeutic levels, dosage may have to be increased when a thiazide is discontinued.

Nonsteroidal anti-inflammatory drugs, such as indomethacin and phenylbutazone, have been reported to reduce lithium clearance and raise serum lithium levels by 25% to 60% (Jefferson et al, 1981; Reimann and Frolich, 1981). It is unknown if other prostaglandin synthesis inhibitors cause a similar action.

Case reports of rare and probably idiosyncratic interactions have been reported with neuroleptics, neuromuscular blocking agents, antibiotics, methyldopa, and digitalis (Jefferson and Marshall, 1981). Definite recommendations await further data.

Before starting lithium   It is important to consider causes of secondary mania. Onset at a late age and the absence of a family history of affective illness should make one suspicious of the presence of a medical cause for mania. Medical causes which have been reported to produce the picture of mania include drugs (including levodopa and steroids), metabolic abnormalities, infection, neoplasm, and temporal lobe epilepsy (Krauthammer and Klerman, 1978).

Mania is also occasionally seen in previously depressed individuals being treated with tricyclic antidepressants or MAOIs. Some researchers feel that this represents the uncovering of an underlying bipolar disorder while others suggest that it is simply a true drug-induced mania.

To rule out secondary mania, a detailed medical history should be supplemented by a physical examination and appropriate laboratory testing. Because of the potential pitfalls involved in treating the manic elderly patient, hospitalization for evaluation and treatment should be strongly considered — particularly if the patient lives alone or has concurrent medical illnesses.

Renal function must be evaluated prior to initiating lithium. Because of the insensitivity of the serum creatinine in the elderly, a 24-hour creatinine clearance is a better test for evaluating GFR. An alternate, but more controversial, method may be to use the formula in chapter 2 to estimate clearance based on serum creatinine, age, weight, and sex.

Thyroid function should be evaluated by measuring serum thyroxine (T_4), L-triodothyronine (T_3), and thyroid-stimulating hormone (TSH). A base-line ECG is mandatory in all elderly patients. Without focal neurologic signs, there is no need to perform a prior EEG or computed tomography (CT) scan (Jefferson, 1983).

Starting lithium   In the elderly it is important to initiate lithium carbonate therapy with a low dose and increase dosage slowly. Liptzin (1984) recommends beginning with a dose of 75 to 300 mg per day while Dunner et al (1979) begin with a 300 mg daily dose of lithium carbonate in all their healthy elderly manics. Doses of 75 mg can be obtained using lithium citrate and doses of 150 mg by breaking a 300 mg tablet in half. Since the elimination half-life of lithium is prolonged in the elderly to as long as 36 hours or more, it may take more than a week to reach steady-state serum levels following either initiation of therapy or a change in dose (Jefferson, 1983).

In elderly manics, more frequent serum levels are generally indicated to minimize the likelihood of toxicity. To appropriately interpret serum lithium levels, they should be drawn 12 hours after the last dose. Unlike most other medications used in psychiatry, the oral dose of lithium is not an adequate guideline and blood levels are crucial for proper management. Therapeutic levels are still not clearly defined in the elderly. In general, they may respond to lower levels than those generally effective in younger patients. Foster and Rosenthal seek blood levels in the range of 0.4 to 0.7 mmol/L and do not exceed 0.7 mmol/L unless a very classic manic picture is present clinically (Foster and Rosenthal, 1980).

Maintenance of lithium   Serum lithium levels and clinical evaluations should be performed more frequently in the elderly as compared to a younger population. If the patient is compliant or is closely watched, he can be evaluated on a monthly basis for the first year of therapy. It is important that the patient and his family be aware of the proper use and toxic side effects and that they are encouraged to contact the physician whenever questions arise. Psychiatrists should have a good working relationship with the patient's internist or general physician.

Side effects and toxicity   Patients with therapeutic levels may complain of tremor, urinary frequency, mild nausea, and a subjective feeling of "being medicated." Early signs of intoxication include increasing tremor, ataxia, weakness, slurred speech, blurred vision, tinnitus, and drowsiness or excitement. Severe intoxication produces increased deep tendon reflexes, nystagmus, confusion, lethargy, and stupor. This may progress to seizures and coma (Table 4-6).

Bradyarrhythmia secondary to sinus node dysfunction occurs uncommonly with lithium therapy (Cassem, 1982). Routine measurement of pulse and asking about typical symptoms such as dizziness or fainting are necessary.

Extrapyramidal effects, particularly parkinsonian movements, have been reported with lithium use and the elderly may be more sensitive to such complications (Jefferson, 1983).

Lithium produces subtle cognitive changes in healthy young volunteers and these may be more marked in the elderly. These can progress to the point where early senile dementia may be suspected (Judd et al, 1977).

Table 4-6
Side Effects of Lithium

Neuromuscular	Nausea
General muscle weakness or	Vomiting
hyperexcitability	Diarrhea
Ataxia	Constipation
Tremor	Dry mouth
Choreoathetotic movements	Metallic taste
Hyperactive reflexes	
	Cardiovascular
Central nervous system	Irregular pulse
Incontinence of urine and feces	Decreased blood pressure
Slurred speech	ECG changes
Blurred vision	Bradycardia
Dizziness	Circulatory collapse
Vertigo	
Seizures	Miscellaneous
Difficulty concentrating	Polyuria
Confusion	Polydipsia
Somnolence or restlessness	Glycosuria
Stupor or coma	Dehydration
	Skin rash
Gastrointestinal	Weight loss or gain
Anorexia	Alopecia

There are reports of acute worsening of eye lens opacification after lithium was started (Makeeva et al, 1974). The number of cases is small and this does not seem to be a common effect. Jefferson states that, at present, lithium use in the elderly is not generally considered reason for periodic eye evaluation (Jefferson, 1983).

The elderly are prone to develop lithium intoxication. They are particularly vulnerable because of reduced lithium clearance secondary to reduced renal function; because of increased sensitivity to the drug, more associated illnesses, multiple medications, poor compliance, decreased food and fluid intake, and lack of social supports. The presence of coexisting neurologic illness is the most critical predisposing factor, according to Himmelhoch and colleagues (Himmelhoch et al, 1980).

Polyuria and polydipsia are so common that they can be considered routine. Thiazide diuretics can be used to decrease these symptoms when they are severe. The mechanism of this paradoxical response to diuretics remains unclear.

Propranolol hydrochloride in small doses (10 to 30 mg/d) may be used to treat lithium-induced tremor. Because propranolol may produce worsening of cardiovascular status and induce depression, it should be used at the lowest possible dose (Liptzin, 1984).

Psychostimulants

Psychostimulants were used briefly as antidepressants until the advent of the tricyclics; at which time the latter became the first line of drugs in the treatment of depression (Myerson, 1936). Nonetheless, recent studies advocating their use in medically ill depressed patients (Kayton and Raskind, 1980; Hackett, 1978; Kaufmann et al, 1984), as adjuvants to morphine in the treatment of postoperative pain (Forest, 1977), and for adjustment reactions in patients recovering from chronic illnesses or surgical procedures (Hackett, 1978), have rekindled interest in the investigation of these agents. Silberman and coworkers (1981), in a double-blind study of 18 endogenously depressed patients, demonstrated superiority of amphetamine over placebo in improving mood and psychomotor activity. Two studies have shown the effectiveness of methylphenidate hydrochloride in treating depressive symptoms in patients with concurrent dementia. In the first study (Holliday and Joffe, 1965), depressed patients with dementia responded better to methylphenidate than to the tricyclic antidepressant protriptyline. In the second (Kaplitz, 1975), methylphenidate was clearly superior to placebo in a double-blind 8-week study; and the methylphenidate group was free of significant side effects. Kaufmann and colleagues (Kaufmann et al, 1984) have reported a number of patients with neurologic or medical disease who responded to psychostimulants.

Indications for stimulants Some indications for stimulants are listed in Table 4-7 (Kaufmann et al, 1982; Kaufmann 1982). At our hospital, stimulants such as methylphenidate or dextroamphetamine are frequently used to treat medically ill or postoperative elderly patients who are apathetic, withdrawn, or depressed. The following case is illustrative.

Case: Mrs A is a 78-year-old woman who became profoundly psychomotorically retarded after gallbladder surgery. She was uncooperative, refused to eat or drink, and stated that she wanted to be left alone to die. A psychiatric consultant recommended methylphenidate 10 mg twice daily. The day after this was begun she brightened considerably, ate and drank on her own, and even walked the corridor a few times. Methylphenidate was discontinued six days later and she was discharged from the hospital 12 days after her operation in good spirits.

Table 4-7
Indications for Psychostimulants

1. Medically ill, apathetic, weakened patients, in whom depression may be easily masked by their concomitant illness

2. To facilitate the rehabilitation process in elderly patients with chronic illnesses, in whom poor compliance with ambulation requirements is frequently due to fatigue, lack of motivation, or anergia

3. Patients with dementia and coexistent retarded/depressive and/or abulic features

4. When electroconvulsive therapy is contraindicated or administratively difficult to perform; eg, if the patient is living in a nursing home

5. Depression with symptoms such as apathy, withdrawn behavior, dysphoria, decreased energy, loss of interest, and poor appetite

Adapted from Kaufmann et al (1984).

We also frequently find that stimulants are helpful for patients with abulia secondary to frontal lobe disease or in demented patients with coexistent retarded-depressive features. The following is an example of such a case (Kaufman et al, 1984).

Case: Mr. B, a 70-year-old retired male who lived with his three sisters, was admitted to our inpatient psychiatric service because of increasing depression. He had no prior psychiatric history. During the year prior to admission, he stayed in bed most of the time with lack of interest in all activities. Approximately three months prior to admission, he began to experience dysphoria, but was not aware of any precipitating events. He denied suicidal ideation, but complained of anorexia with a 20-lb weight loss and noted a need for more sleep. He also suffered from persistent fatigue, decreased energy, and constipation. About one month prior to admission, he started to urinate and move his bowels in bed. For the two weeks before hospitalization, he refused to move or get out of bed. His sisters arranged for admission to a neurology service where a complete neurologic and metabolic workup was negative except for clinical signs of recent memory impairment, poor concentration, episodic disorientation, and the CT scan which revealed marked frontal and temporal lobe atrophy. He was treated with doxepin up to 200 mg daily and transferred to our psychiatric unit with diagnoses of organic brain disease and retarded depression. After lack of significant improvement on doxepin, concurrent with some further deterioration of cognitive function as the dose was being raised, the medication was discontinued. He was then given a full course of electroconvulsive therapy (ECT) which normalized his eating and sleeping patterns. However, he remained dysphoric, abulic, and refused to get out of bed or even to wash and care for himself. A trial of low dose haloperidol produced no improvement. While nursing home placement was being considered, a trial of methylphenidate 5 mg three times a day was started. Results were dramatic. The morning after methylphenidate was started, he got out of bed and washed and shaved himself. For the first time since admission, he started several conversations with patients, his mood became brighter, and he approached his ward physician with questions about discharge. This improvement persisted throughout the remainder of his hospitalization. However, the impairment in his cognitive functions, associated with chronic organic brain disease, did not improve. Nonetheless, he was discharged to his home. On six-month follow-up, there had been no relapse of depression, and he continued to take methylphenidate 5 mg three times a day with no side effects.

Alternatives to tricyclic antidepressants may be necessary in the treatment of depression in medically ill patients. The development of confusional states secondary to anticholinergic side effects and excessive sedation of some antidepressants has been discussed. Depressed patients with structurally compromised brain function who are undergoing treatment with tricyclic antidepressants may have a deficit of acetylcholine, and therefore may be especially vulnerable to these adverse reactions (Crook and Cohen, 1981).

Psychostimulants may exert their antidepressant effects by blocking reuptake of catecholamines, thus prolonging the effects of synaptically released dopamine and norepinephrine (Brown, 1977).

Hackett has described the usefulness of psychostimulants in diagnosing and effectively treating medically ill apathetic weakened patients in whom depression might be easily masked by their concomitant illness (Hackett, 1978). The rapid improvement in the physical and psychological symptomatology speeds up the recovery, in some cases dramatically. This rapid response to treatment, usually within 24 to 48 hours, is of additional benefit for this type of patient, since concurrent medical illness makes it more of a hazard to wait ten to 14 days for the tricyclic antidepressants to become clinically effective.

The therapeutic use of amphetamine and methylphenidate for depression may not be legal in some jurisdictions, and not considered acceptable in others. It is tempting to speculate from previous studies (Forest, 1977; Holliday and Joffe, 1965; Kaplitz, 1975; Myerson, 1936; Katon and Raskind, 1980) that there is a wide margin of safety between therapeutic and toxic doses where unwanted physical and psychological side effects may appear. Further well-designed clinical studies are warranted to confirm these observations.

Table 4-8
Drug Interactions with Stimulants

Drug	Effect
Guanethidine	Decreases hypotensive effects
Vasopressors	Increase pressor effect
Oral anticoagulants	Increase prothrombin time (methylphenidate only)
Phenobarbital, phenytoin, primidone	Increases anticonvulsant blood levels
Imipramine, desipramine	Increases antidepressant blood levels

Dosage and monitoring   Dextroamphetamine is roughly twice as potent as methylphenidate. Therapeutic effects are usually achieved with daily doses of 20 to 40 mg of methylphenidate or 10 to 20 mg of dextroamphetamine given orally in two divided doses, preferably 30 minutes before meals (Kaufmann, 1982). It is best to administer the last dose before 4 PM in order to avoid insomnia. If there is no therapeutic response in 48 to 72 hours, the medication should be discontinued. Occasionally, patients may develop some emotional lability, at which point the dose may be reduced to 10 mg daily.

The duration of treatment is usually empirical and individualized to the clinical situation (Kaufmann, 1982; Kaufmann et al, 1984). For example, if the onset of depressive symptoms is recent, of moderate intensity, and associated with a concurrent medical illness, the stimulant might be needed for only one or two weeks. In other cases, if the symptoms are progressing in severity or there has been a relapse, treatment may be necessary for a few months.

Although no clinically significant alterations in blood, serum, or urinary parameters occur at therapeutic dosages, during prolonged therapy it is recommended that routine laboratory tests be performed on a regular basis. Vital signs, especially blood pressure, should be monitored in hypertensive patients (Kaufmann, 1982). Common drug interactions are listed in Table 4-8.

The response to methylphenidate in many patients illustrates three important issues: (1) the quick remission of symptoms following a small dose of stimulant; (2) the lack of toxic side effects; (3) no recurrence of symptoms after stimulant was discontinued. Although stimulants are not a panacea, there are specific indications for their short-term use.

POSTSTROKE DEPRESSION

Each year 440,000 people have thromboembolic strokes in the United States (Wolf et al, 1977). Between 30% and 60% of poststroke patients have clinically important depressions and the period of high risk lasts for two years poststroke (Robinson, 1981; Lipsey et al, 1984).

Depressions reportedly occur more often in patients suffering right, rather than left, hemisphere strokes. Robinson and colleagues concluded from animal studies that brain catecholamines are depleted in cerebrovascular accidents, and suggested that antidepressant medications might be used to treat these conditions (Robinson et al, 1983; Robinson and Szetela, 1981).

There are case reports that psychostimulants may be useful in stroke-induced depressions (Kaufmann et al, 1984; Robinson, 1981). They may exert their antidepressant effects by blocking the reuptake of depleted catecholamines.

A recent study by Lipsey et al (1984) showed that the tricyclic nortriptyline significantly improved poststroke depression when compared in a double-blind manner to placebo. Successfully treated patients had nortriptyline levels in the therapeutic range (50 to 150 ng/mL). Because the number of patients in this study was small (34) they were unable to determine the relationship between lesion location and response to medication. The demonstration by Lipsey et al of the success of nortriptyline in the treatment of poststroke depression represents a potentially important advance in the treatment of stroke patients. Certainly, stroke patients have many difficulties dealing with issues of rehabilitation and should not be forced to suffer concomitant depression when we have the tools at hand to effectively treat such symptoms.

CARDIAC PATIENTS

Many clinicians avoid the use of antidepressants in elderly patients with cardiac disease. Physicians probably allow many moderately severe depressions to go untreated because of unwarranted fears about the cardiac side effects of antidepressants. Cassem (1982) reviewed the relevant issues in detail and concluded that when certain precautions are taken, antidepressants can generally be safely used even in very ill cardiac patients.

There are four main side effects that are of particular concern in using antidepressants in cardiac patients: (1) orthostatic hypotension, (2) anticholinergic effects, (3) cardiac conduction effects, and (4) decreased cardiac contractility. These will be reviewed individually.

Orthostatic Hypotension

Postural changes in blood pressure occur commonly with antidepressant agents. Tertiary amine tricyclics (amitriptyline, imipramine, doxepin) tend to cause more severe hypotensive effects than secondary amines (nortriptyline, desipramine). With tricyclics, the best clinical predictor of drug-induced postural hypotension is the predrug orthostatic fall in blood pressure. Cassem (1982) estimates that in patients with a mean predrug fall in lying-to-standing systolic blood pressure of 10 mmHg, the mean orthostatic change on imipramine will be about 25 mmHg. It is not known whether such predrug conclusions can be drawn for the newer nontricyclic antidepressants or for the MAOIs. The newer agents such as amoxapine, maprotiline, and trazodone appear to offer no advantage in avoiding orthostatic hypotension (Cassem, 1982).

Orthostatic hypotension is one of the primary side effects of MAOIs. It is not felt to be dose-dependent and has usually been described as an early side effect. That is, it was felt that if patients tolerated the first few days of medication, then hypotension would rarely necessitate stopping the drug. As noted earlier, however, recent data indicate that these concepts may be in error. Kronig and associates (Kronig et al, 1983) studied 14 patients with a mean age of 52 who were treated with phenelzine and found that the mean orthostatic drop increased with time in a generally linear fashion. The maximum mean orthostatic drop was 12 mmHg at week 4. It appears, from their data, that the elderly were no more likely to have severe orthostatic changes than were younger patients. The consequences, however, of a fall in blood pressure in an old person are much more likely to be serious.

Lithium therapy is not associated with orthostatic hypotension.

Anticholinergic Effects

Anticholinergic effects are particularly toxic for elderly patients. Anticholinergic potency can be quantified (Table 4-9) (Snyder and Yamamura, 1974; Richelson, 1982).

All of the available tricyclic antidepressants have significant anticholinergic effects. The main cardiac effect of most concern is tachycardia. In general, tertiary amines are more potent anticholinergic agents than secondary amines, with amitriptyline significantly exceeding all other tricyclics (Cassem, 1982) with the possible exception of protriptyline (Tollefson et al, 1982). Recent data indicate that protriptyline may be the worst offender in this class of drugs. Cassem (1982) still regards amitriptyline as the tricyclic agent most likely to cause a clinically hazardous tachycardia. Those cardiac patients with ischemic disease are least able to tolerate an increase in heart rate.

Amoxapine and maprotiline offer little improvement over earlier tricyclics in terms of anticholinergic properties. Trazodone, however, has no anticholinergic effects and may be useful in patients at risk from tachycardia.

One great advantage of the MAOIs is their essential lack of anticholinergic side effects (Table 4-9) (Jenike, 1984b). No regular changes in cardiac rhythm have been associated with the MAOIs, even in cases of overdose.

Lithium also has no anticholinergic effects and does not produce tachycardia (Cassem, 1982).

Decreased Contractility

It is a frequent fear that tricyclics may induce congestive heart failure because of their negative ionotropic effect. In reviewing the data, Cassem (1982) noted that most studies employed indirect measurements of cardiac function, such as systolic time intervals, which could have reflected slowing of H-V conduction commonly produced by tricyclics rather than decreased contractility. Veith et al (1982) using radionuclide

Table 4-9
Anticholinergic Potency of Some Psychotropic Agents

Agent	Richelson (1982)*	Snyder and Yamamura (1977)†
Atropine	55	0.4
Trihexyphenidyl (Artane)	—	0.6
Benztropine (Cogentin)	—	1.5
Amitriptyline (Elavil)	5.5	10
Protriptyline (Vivactil)	4.0	—
Doxepin (Sinequan)	1.3	44
Imipramine (Tofranil)	1.1	78
Nortriptyline (Aventyl)	0.7	—
Desipramine (Norpramin)	0.5	170
Maprotiline (Ludiomil)	0.2	—
Amoxapine (Ascendin)	0.1	—
Trazodone (Desyrel)	0.003	—
Phenelzine (Nardil)	—	100,000

*The larger the number, the greater the anticholinergic effect.
†The smaller the number, the greater the anticholinergic effect.

ventriculograms to measure ejection fractions before and during max-imum exercise in depressed patients with heart disease on therapeutic doses of imipramine and doxepin, demonstrated no adverse effects on left ventricular function.

Glassman and colleagues (1983) also studied a group of depressed patients with clinically significant pre-existing left ventricular dysfunc-tion by means of radionuclide angiography. Of 15 patients in their study, 13 had ejection fraction values that were more than two stan-dard deviations below normal controls. They found that therapeutic levels of imipramine did not further impair left ventricular performance and that ejection fraction was unchanged during treatment.

There is also no evidence that the newer nontricyclic agents, lithium, or the MAOIs affect cardiac contractility.

Cardiac Conduction Effects

The tricyclics slow conduction in the His bundle and Purkinje fibers and can exacerbate pre-existing ventricular conduction deficits (Rudorfer and Young, 1980). The ECG manifestations include increased PR, QRS, and QTc intervals as well as a decrease in T-wave amplitude (Cassem, 1982). This effect appears to be correlated with anticholiner-gic activity with trazodone causing the least slowing (Gomoll and Byrne, 1979; Hayes et al, 1983).

The risk of worsening cardiac arrhythmias with antidepressant ther-apy has been overemphasized in the past since imipramine and prob-ably the other tricyclic antidepressants are actually effective antiarrhythmic agents, similar in action to group I agents like quini-dine and procainamide (Giardina et al, 1979). In fact, patients on quini-dine or procainamide should be followed carefully, and their antiarrhythmic medication may need to be reduced when a tricyclic an-tidepressant is added. Studies documenting the antiarrhythmic efficacy of imipramine and nortriptyline (Giardina et al, 1981) can be shared with colleagues who may be reluctant to use antidepressants in patients with arrhythmias.

It is important to note that there is no relationship between the initial PR and QRS intervals and the drug-related change after starting imipramine (Giardina et al, 1979). That is, patients with a pre-existing prolonged PR or QRS interval do not have any greater changes than those with an initially short PR or QRS interval.

Clinical problems associated with slowed conduction are rare. Giardina et al (1979) found that none of 14 patients with conduction abnormalities developed second-degree heart block. Of the 14 patients, five had first-degree heart block and five had right bundle-branch block. Of those patients who overdose on tricyclics, only 6% to 20% develop significant clinical problems with conduction abnormalities (Biggs et al, 1977; Callahan, 1979).

It has been demonstrated that increases in PR and QRS intervals are directly related to tricyclic plasma levels (Giardina et al, 1979), and ECGs can provide a reliable guide to the cardiac effects of the tricyclic as dose is increased. In cases of severe conduction abnormalities, such as sick sinus syndrome, Cassem (1982) recommends pacemaker protection from complete heart block.

There are case reports that both amoxapine and maprotiline have been associated with arrhythmias (Cassem, 1982; Zavodnick, 1981). Trazodone is generally free of clinical conduction problems in healthy individuals, but has been associated with arrhythmias in patients with pre-existing cardiac illness. There are no consistent changes in cardiac rhythm associated with the MAOIs, even in cases of overdosage (Cassem, 1982).

Lithium regularly produces T-wave flattening in about 50% of the ECGs of patients with drug levels over 0.5 mmol/L (Jefferson and Greist, 1977). These changes may be secondary to altered ionic equilibrium with intracellular hypokalemia. Potassium is normal in these cases. Toxic cardiac effects are uncommon, but reversible sinus node abnormalities and other conduction disturbances have been reported (Wellens et al, 1975; Wilson et al, 1976; Jaffe, 1977). Cassem (1982) recommends that patients with pre-existing cardiac conduction abnormalities be given continuous cardiac monitoring during the initiation of lithium therapy.

Patients with heart disease can generally be managed on antidepressant medication. Any patients with heart disease should be followed with frequent ECGs. Inquiry about cardiac symptoms such as ankle edema, dyspnea on exertion, orthopnea, and paroxysmal nocturnal dyspnea should be done at each visit. The patients should be examined for rales and the presence of changing heart sounds.

POTENTIATION OF ANTIDEPRESSANT EFFECTS BY LITHIUM OR THYROID HORMONE

As noted earlier, lithium may be a useful adjuvant in tricyclic antidepressant-resistant unipolar depression. DeMontigny and associates reported that eight such patients (aged 33 to 64) responded within 48 hours after low-dose lithium was added to the tricyclic regimen (deMontigny et al, 1981). In addition, Louie and Meltzer (1984) reported on nine patients who were unresponsive to antidepressants alone who were given lithium carbonate to potentiate the antidepressant. Two of their patients showed sustained improvement, two showed transient improvement but then relapsed, two other cases with bipolar histories became manic, and three did not respond. In their study, the time between lithium addition and improvement of depressive symptoms was frequently longer than deMontigny et al reported and ranged from two to 12 days.

L-Triiodothyronine (T_3) has also been reported to potentiate the effect of the tricyclics. Goodwin et al (1982) reported on six women and six men who were treated in a double-blind fashion for major depressive illness which did not respond to imipramine or amitriptyline, 150 to 300 mg/d, during periods ranging from 26 to 112 days. After the addition of 25 ug/d (ten patients) or 50 ug/d (two patients) of T_3, nine patients showed statistically significant improvement in depression scores; in eight the response was marked. Improvement generally began within one to three days and was noted in all aspects of the depressive syndrome. Side effects were minimal and T_3 did not change plasma levels of imipramine or desipramine or their ratio but did suppress thyroxine. The work of Goodwin et al followed earlier uncontrolled reports of T_3 acceleration of response to tricyclic antidepressants; five studies suggested that some depressed patients who were not responsive to tricyclics became responders when T_3 was added (Earle, 1970; Ogura et al, 1974; Banki, 1975; 1977; Tsutsui et al, 1979).

These adjuvants may be particularly helpful in treatment-resistant patients. Despite the well-established efficacy of tricyclic antidepressant agents (Baldessarini, 1977), controlled studies indicate that the rate of nonresponse or partial response is in the range of 20% to 35% (Goodwin et al, 1982; Klein and Davis, 1969). Goodwin and colleagues went so far in their report to suggest that a trial of a tricyclic antidepressant in a depressed patient should not be considered a failure until T_3 potentiation has been tried.

ELECTROCONVULSIVE THERAPY

Electroconvulsive therapy (ECT), as practiced today, is the electrical induction of a series of grand mal seizures, usually six to ten, in patients with susceptible psychiatric disorders, primarily severe depression. The seizure itself, rather than the electrical stimulus, is the therapeutic agent. The technique of ECT has been refined over the past few decades, and today the use of anticholinergic premedication, short-acting barbiturates for anesthesia, muscle relaxants, oxygenation, low-energy stimulus wave forms, and unilateral stimulus electrode placement have all acted to decrease the risks and side effects without diminishing its therapeutic efficacy (Jenike, 1983h; 1984c; Weiner, 1982).

Electroconvulsive therapy is typically given every other day, three times a week, in order to minimize brain dysfunction. If there is significant confusion, memory loss, or behavior change, all of which tend to increase with the number of treatments, the interval between treatments may be extended.

When it was initially introduced in 1938, ECT represented the first line of treatment, not only for depression but also for schizophrenia (Weiner, 1982). With the advent of antidepressant medication in the 1950s, the use of ECT began to decline. Although these drugs are not as effective as ECT, they are more convenient and do not involve a procedure whose mere mention can be frightening to many patients and their families. During the last decade, the use of ECT has stabilized at approximately 80,000 patients per year in this country (Electroconvulsive Therapy, American Psychiatric Association Task Force on ECT, 1978).

Electroconvulsive therapy may be the only choice of treatment in the elderly depressed patient whose illness is accompanied by self-destructive behavior, such as suicide attempts or refusal to eat. In these cases, a drug trial lasting four to six weeks may be associated with significant risk. In these patients, ECT, which characteristically begins to exert significant beneficial effects within the first week, may be dramatically lifesaving.

Depression is common in all age groups, but ECT is used to a greater extent in the elderly. This is because depression is more likely to be severe in the older patient, and also because the elderly are more likely to suffer from concurrent chronic diseases for which the antidepressant drugs may be less desirable due to their anticholinergic, cardiotoxic, and hypotensive effects (Weiner, 1982).

Electroconvulsive therapy is both more effective and faster-acting than drugs in the treatment of depression. Many depressed elderly patients, especially those with psychotic symptoms, do not respond to drugs but do respond to ECT. In one study, for example, remission occurred in 80% to 85% of drug nonresponders (Scovern and Kilmann, 1980). Electroconvulsive therapy has consistently outperformed tricyclic antidepressants and MAOIs with 10% to 20% more patients showing improvement. Not only is ECT more effective than pharmacologic agents, but it may be safer for those patients with serious illness, particularly that involving cardiac dysfunction.

Risks and Side Effects

The mortality with the use of ECT has been estimated at around 1/10,000 patients, which is probably considerably less than that associated with any of the drugs indicated in the treatment of depression (Fink, 1979; Weiner, 1982). Clinically, ECT is commonly associated with confusion and temporary amnesia, and physiologically, by slowing on EEG. Even though some patients complain of mild memory loss for months or even years after receiving ECT, objective memory testing in such cases does not appear to bear out the presence of an organic defect. No studies have documented any significant irreversible pathologic changes in the brain (Weiner, 1982). Most ECT patients do not consider themselves affected by persistent memory deficits, and they tend to view their treatments as no more upsetting than a visit to the dentist (Hughes et al, 1981).

Insulin-dependent diabetes mellitus is reportedly more difficult to control when diabetic patients are concomitantly depressed (Kronfol et al, 1981; Crammer and Gillies, 1981). If insulin levels are adjusted upward while a patient is depressed, sugars should be carefully monitored during and after treatment of the depression. The following case report describes an elderly insulin-dependent diabetic woman who had significantly lowered blood sugars after ECT (Normand and Jenike, 1984, reproduced with permission).

> *Case:* A 73-year-old woman with a 20-year history of insulin-dependent diabetes mellitus was admitted to our inpatient psychiatric service for treatment of a psychotic depression. She was suffering from insomnia, decreased appetite with a 10 pound weight loss in the last few months, agitation, and paranoia. She believed that her food was being poisoned and that she was being punished for past sins. She had recently been treated with maprotiline, thiothixene, and lithium citrate without effect. Her history included three episodes of depression (the last one three years prior to this admission) which were clinically similar to the present episode and did not respond to medication but did resolve completely after ECT.
>
> On this admission she refused ECT and thus guardianship proceedings were begun. She consumed a 1500-calorie diet (American Diabetic Association) throughout this hospitalization. Blood sugar levels remained above 80 mg/dL for the next two weeks prior to starting ECT, on 15 to 30 units of NPH insulin each morning. Two weeks after admission, ECT was begun and administered at most every other day until six treatments had been given. She received 20 units NPH and 5 units regular insulin on each day that she did not receive ECT. Since she was given nothing by mouth on ECT mornings, the insulin dose was lowered to 10 units NPH in the morning with 5 units in the afternoon on days she received ECT.

Her mood improved markedly and the delusions abated; however, she was intermittently confused and disoriented. The confusion was initially attributed to the ECT, but two blood sugar levels measured between the fourth and fifth ECT treatments were at 78 and 58 mg/dL — lower than any pre-ECT levels at our hospital. Insulin was discontinued and over the next three days the sugar levels remained between 100 to 200 mg/dL with only 5 units of regular insulin each afternoon. Her confusion resolved despite another ECT treatment. Over the next week, the sugar levels gradually rose to almost 400 mg/dL and insulin was restarted. A few weeks later she was discharged euthymic on 15 units NPH insulin each morning with well-controlled sugar levels.

There are earlier reports of elderly depressed patients whose blood sugars fell after ECT and one group (Fakhri et al, 1980; Fakhri, 1966) even suggested that ECT may be a cure for diabetes mellitus. In all of the diabetics that responded to ECT, however, the diabetes was of recent onset and noninsulin-dependent. All of Fakhri's patients were depressed clinically and the primary indication for ECT was treatment of the depression. It is now well documented (Carroll et al, 1981; Jenike, 1982c) that many endogenously depressed nondiabetic patients have abnormally high plasma cortisol concentrations 24 hours after a dose of dexamethasone. These patients also have high concentrations of ACTH and corticosteroids (Butler and Besser, 1968; Sachar et al, 1973). Recently, Jenike (1982c) theorized that perhaps Fakhri's "diabetics" who responded to ECT were actually endogenously depressed and that their hyperglycemia and glycosuria were secondary to the diabetogenic effects of increased ACTH and corticosteroids. It has been shown that after ECT, the ACTH and corticosteroid levels return to normal, which may in time bring the blood glucose level back to normal and could account for the amelioration of the apparent diabetes. Kronfol and associates alternatively suggest that the blood sugar level may be driven up in depression by elevated levels of growth hormone, an insulin antagonist (Kronfol et al, 1981). Baldessarini (1981), however, described conflicting results from different studies on growth hormone levels in depression. The Kronfol group also wondered if increased epinephrine secretion in depression could account for insulin resistance; however, Crammer and Gillies (1981) measured urinary vanillylmandelic acid excretion (a measure of peripheral epinephrine turnover) on two occasions in one patient and it was normal. Even though the mechanisms remain speculative, the weight of the evidence indicates that the blood sugar levels and insulin requirements of depressed insulin-dependent diabetics are lowered after a course of ECT. *If the blood sugar levels are not carefully monitored and the insulin dosage reduced accordingly, the levels may become dangerously low, producing a clinical picture that may resemble the mental status changes frequently occurring after ECT.*

In ECT therapy, it is the electrical stimulus, not the seizure itself, that is the component most responsible for the side effects of confusion and transient loss of memory. A recent study involving 29 patients (mean age 73) showed that electrical stimuli given only over the nondominant hemisphere produced therapeutic results comparable to bilateral stimulation (Fraser and Glass, 1978; Fraser and Glass, 1980). The degree of postictal confusion, however, was much greater for those receiving bilateral ECT, indicating that the acute cerebral impairment was less in those patients who received unilateral, nondominant stimulation.

Even though there are really no absolute contraindications to ECT, there are certain conditions in which a marked increase in associated morbidity and mortality may be seen (Electroconvulsive Therapy, American Psychiatric Association Task Force on ECT, 1978; Fink, 1979). These include recent myocardial infarction or stroke, severe hypertension, and the presence of an intracerebral mass. In these patients, ECT should generally be delayed until effective medical management has been initiated or until adequate recovery time has elapsed. If ECT is urgently indicated, however, appropriate premedication and close monitoring can help to minimize the risk.

SUMMARY

Depression is a common debilitating and often life-threatening illness in the elderly. We have reviewed diagnosis, medical assessment, and evaluation of suicide potential. The potential usefulness of the DST has been covered and an analogy to the ESR is presented. In the absence of either medical illness or medication that affects the DST, resistance to dexamethasone suppression strongly suggests the presence of a major depressive disorder. A normal DST does not, however, rule out such a disorder. Mild to moderate dementia may not invalidate the DST as a clinical aid in detecting depression.

Drug treatment of depression is reviewed. Tertiary amines cause significant orthostatic hypotension and probably should be avoided in the elderly. Amitriptyline, and possibly protriptyline, are extremely anticholinergic and are best avoided. Amoxapine is essentially a neuroleptic with some antidepressant properties and may induce neurologic sequelae including tardive dyskinesia.

If a patient has had a prior positive response or if he has a relative who had a good outcome from a particular drug, it may be best to begin treatment with this drug. The choice of antidepressant can be based largely on the clinical picture. For example, if a depressed patient is sleeping much more than usual and requires an activating (noradrenergic) agent, desipramine would be a good drug to try. If, on the other hand, the patient is unable to sleep, a more sedating agent like nortriptyline or trazodone should be tried. Risks and side effects, as well as use in cardiac patients, are reviewed in detail. Management of overdoses is reviewed.

Many clinicians avoid the use of MAOIs in the elderly patient because of fear of adverse reactions. This fear is largely unfounded. Precautions, side effects, and specific recommendations are outlined.

Using lithium in the elderly requires some special precautions because of decreased GFR and potential interactions with concomitantly used drugs. Side effects and toxicity are discussed.

The usage of psychostimulants, such as methylphenidate and amphetamine, to treat medically ill depressed patients is reviewed. These agents are also sometimes useful in demented individuals or in patients with abulic frontal lobe syndromes.

Poststroke depressions are common and recent evidence indicates that they can be adequately treated. Stroke patients have many difficulties dealing with issues of rehabilitation and should not be forced to suffer concomitant depression when we have the tools at hand to effectively treat such symptoms.

Recent data on the potentiation of antidepressant effects by lithium or T_3 indicate that they may possibly be useful in some tricyclic-resistant patients.

Risks, side effects, and recent procedural advances in the use of ECT are reviewed. Electroconvulsive therapy is both more effective and faster-acting than drugs in the treatment of depression. Many depressed elderly patients, especially those with psychotic symptoms, do not respond to drugs but improve drastically with ECT.

REFERENCES

Amsterdam JD, Winokur A, Caroff SN, et al: The dexamethasone suppression test in outpatients with primary affective disorder and healthy control subjects. *Am J Psychiatry* 139(3):287–291, 1982.

Anderson WH: Depression, in Lazare A (ed): *Outpatient Psychiatry*. Baltimore, Williams & Wilkins, pp 257–260, 1979.

Angst J, Baastrup P, Grof P, et al: The course of monopolar depression and bipolar psychoses. *Psychiatr Neurol Neurochir* 76:489–500, 1973.

Anonymous: Psychiatric illness among medical patients. *Lancet* 1:479, 1979.

Arana GW, Barreira PJ, Cohen BJ, et al: The dexamethasone suppression test in mania, schizophrenia, and other psychotic disorders. *Am J Psychiatry* 140:1521-1523, 1983.

Ashford W, Ford CV: Use of MAO inhibitors in elderly patients. *Am J Psychiatry* 136:1466, 1979.

Avery D, Winokur G: Mortality in depressed patients treated with electroconvulsive therapy and antidepressants. *Arch Gen Psychiatry* 33:1029-1937, 1976.

Baldessarini RJ: *Chemotherapy in Psychiatry*. Cambridge, Mass, Harvard University Press, 1977.

Baldessarini RJ: A summary of biomedical aspects of mood disorders. *McLean Hosp J* 6:1-34, 1981.

Banki CM: Triiodothyronine in the treatment of depression. *Orv Hetil* 116:2543-2546, 1975.

Banki CM: Cerebrospinal fluid amine metabolites after combined amitriptyline-triiodothyronine treatment of depressed women. *Eur J Pharmacol* 11:311-315, 1977.

Barton JL: Amoxapine-induced agitation among bipolar depressed patients. *Am J Psychiatry* 139:387, 1982.

Biggs JT, Spiker DG, Petit JM, et al: Tricyclic antidepressant overdose. *JAMA* 238:135-138, 1977.

Brooks SM, Werk EE, Ackerman SJ, et al: Adverse effects of phenobarbital on corticosteroid metabolism in patients with bronchial asthma. *N Engl J Med* 286:1125-1128, 1972.

Brown WA: Psychologic and neuroendocrine responses to methylphenidate. *Arch Gen Psychiatry* 34:1103-1108, 1977.

Brown WA: The dexamethasone suppression test: Clinical applications. *Psychosomatics* 22(11):951-955, 1981.

Brown WA, Johnson R, Mayfield D: The 24-hour dexamethasone suppression test in a clinical setting: Relationship to diagnosis, symptoms, and response to treatment. *Am J Psychiatry* 136:543-547, 1979.

Butler PW, Besser GM: Pituitary-adrenal function in severe depressive illness. *Lancet* 1:1234-1236, 1968.

Cade R, Shires DL, Barrow NV, et al: Abnormal diurnal variation of plasma cortisol in patients with renovascular hypertension. *J Clin Endocrinol Metab* 27:800-806, 1976.

Callahan M: Tricyclic antidepressant overdose. *JACEP* 8:413-425, 1979.

Carroll BJ: The hypothalamic-pituitary-adrenal axis in depression, in Davies B, Carroll BJ, Mowbray RM (eds): *Depressive Illness, Some Research Studies*. Springfield, Ill, Charles C Thomas, 1972.

Carroll BJ: Neuroendocrine function in psychiatric disorders, in Lipton MA, DiMascio A, Killam DR (eds): *Psychopharmacology: A Generation of Progress*. New York, Raven Press, 1978, pp 487-496.

Carroll BJ, Curtis GC, Mendels J: Neuroendocrine regulation in depression: II Discrimination of depressed from nondepressed patients. *Arch Gen Psychiatry* 33:1051-1058, 1976.

Carroll BJ, Feinberg M, Greden JF, et al: A specific laboratory test for the diagnosis of melancholia. *Arch Gen Psychiatry* 38:15-22, 1981.

Cassem NH: Cardiovascular effects of antidepressants. *J Clin Psychiatry* 43:11(sect 2):22-28, 1982.

Clayton PJ: Mortality and morbidity in the first year of widowhood. *Arch Gen Psychiatry* 30: 747–750, 1974.

Cole JO, Branconnier R, Salomon M, et al: Tricyclic use in the cognitively impaired elderly. *J Clin Psychiatry* September(Sec 2):14–19, 1983.

Crammer J. Gillis C: Psychiatric aspects of diabetes mellitus: Diabetes and depression. *Br J Psychiatry* 139:171–172, 1981.

Crook T, Cohen GD (eds): *Physicians' Handbook on Psychotherapeutic Drug Use in the Aged.* New Canaan, Conn, Mark Powley Associates, 1981.

Davidson J, White H: The effect of isocarboxazid on platelet MAO activity. *Biol Psychiatry* 18:1075–1079, 1983.

Dec GW, Jenike MA, Stern TA: Trazodone-digoxin interaction in an animal model. *J Clin Psychopharmacol* 4:153–155, 1984.

deMontigny C, Grunberg F, Mayer A, et al: Lithium induces rapid relief of depression in tricyclic antidepressant drug non-responders. *Br J Psychiatry* 138:252–256, 1981.

Dewan M, Pandurangi AK, Boucher ML, et al: Abnormal dexamethasone suppression test results in chronic schizophrenic patients. *Am J Psychiatry* 139:1501–1503, 1982.

Dominquez RA: Evaluating the effectiveness of the new antidepressants. *Hosp Community Psychiatry* 34:405–407, 1983.

Dunner DL, Roose SP, Bone S: Complications of lithium treatment in older patients, in Geshon S; Kline NS, Shou M, (eds): *Lithium Controversies and Unresolved Issues.* Amsterdam, Excerpta Medica, 1979, pp 427–431.

Earle BV: Thyroid hormone and tricyclic antidepressants in resistant depressions. *Am J Psychiatry* 126:1667–1669, 1970.

Electroconvulsive Therapy, American Psychiatric Association Task Force on ECT. Task force report No. 14. Washington, DC, American Psychiatric ssociation, 1978.

Elias AN, Gwinup G: Effects of some clinically encountered drugs on steroid and degradation. *Metabolism* 29:582–595, 1980.

Fakhri O: Blood sugar after electroplexy. *Lancet* 1:587, 1966.

Fakhri O, Fadhl AA, el Rawdi RM: Effective electroconvulsive therapy on diabetes mellitus. *Lancet* 11:775–777, 1980.

Feinberg T, Goodman B: Affective illness, dementia, and pseudodementia. *J Clin Psychiatry* 45:99–103, 1984.

Fink M: *Convulsive Therapy: Theory and Practice.* New York, Raven Press, 1979.

Forest WH: Dextroamphetamine with morphine for the treatment of postoperative pain. *N Engl J Med* 296:712–715, 1977.

Foster JR, Rosenthal JS: Lithium treatment of the elderly, in Johnson FN (ed): *Handbook of Lithium Therapy.* Lancaster, England, MTP Press, 1980, pp 414–420.

Fraser RM, Glass IB: Recovery from ECT in elderly patients. *Br J Psychiatry* 133:524, 1978.

Fraser RM, Glass IB: Unilateral and bilateral ECT in elderly patients. *Acta Psychiatr Scand* 62:13, 1980.

Gelenberg AJ: The DST in perspective. *Biol Ther in Psychiatry* 6:1–2, 1983.

Gelenberg AJ: Heterocyclic antidepressant overdose. *Topics in Geriatrics* 2:33–34,36, 1984.

Giardina E-GV, Bigger JT, Glassman AH, et al: The electrocardiographic and antiarrhythmic effects of imipramine hydrochloride at therapeutic plasma concentrations. *Circulation* 60:1045–1052, 1979.

Giardina EGV, Bigger JT, Johnson LL: The effect of imipramine and nortriptyline on ventricular premature depolarizations and left ventricular function. *Circulation* 64:316, 1981.

Glassman AH, Johnson LL, Giardina EGV, et al: The use of imipramine in depressed patients with congestive heart failure. *JAMA* 250:1997–2001, 1983.

Goldberg IK: Dexamethasone suppression test as indicator of safe withdrawal of antidepressant therapy. *Lancet* 2:376, 1980a.

Goldberg IK: Dexamethsone suppression tests in depression and response to treatment. *Lancet* 2:92, 1980b.

Goldberg MJ, Spector R: Amoxapine overdose: Report of two patients with severe neurologic damage. *Ann Intern Med* 96:463–464, 1982.

Gomoll AW, Byrne JE: Trazodone and imipramine: Comparative effects on canine cardiac conduction. *Eur J Pharmacol* 57:335–342, 1979.

Goodman LS, Gilman A: *The Pharmacological Basis of Therapeutics.* New York, MacMillan Publishing Co, Inc, 1975.

Goodwin FK, Prange AJ, Post RM, et al: Potentiation of antidepressant effects of L-triiodothyronine in tricyclic nonresponders. *Am J Psychiatry* 139:34–38, 1982.

Graham PM, Booth J, Boranga E, et al: The dexamethasone suppression in mania. *J Affective Disord* 4:201–211, 1982.

Greden JF, Albala AA, Haskett RF, et al: Normalization of dexamethasone suppression test: A laboratory index of recovery from endogenous depression. *Biol Psychiatry* 15:449–458, 1980.

Greden JF, Carroll BJ: The dexamethasone suppression test as a diagnostic aid in catatonia. *Am J Psychiatry* 136:1199–1200, 1979.

Guggenheim FG: Suicide, in Hackett TP, Cassem NH (eds): *Massachusetts General Hospital Handbook of General Hospital Psychiatry.* St. Louis, CV Mosby, 1978, pp 250–263.

Gurland BJ: The comparative frequency of depression in various adult age groups. *J Gerontol* 31:283–292, 1976.

Hackett TP: *The Use of Stimulant Drugs in General Hospital Psychiatry,* tape. Glendale Calif, Audio-Digest Foundation, Vol 7(12), 1978.

Hayes RL, Gerner RH, Fairbanks L, et al: EKG findings in geriatric depressives given trazodone, placebo or imipramine. *J Clin Psychiatry* 44:180–183, 1983.

Himmelhoch JM: Cardiovascular effects of trazodone in humans. *J Clin Psychopharmacol* 1(65):765–815, 1981.

Himmelhoch JM, Neil JF, May SJ, et al: Age, dementia, dyskinesias, and lithium response. *Am J Psychiatry* 137:941–945, 1980.

Holliday AR, Joffe JR: A controlled evaluation of protriptyline compared to placebo and to methylphenidate hydrochloride. *J New Drugs* 5:257, 1965.

Hughes J, Barraclough BM, Reeve W: Are patients shocked by ECT? *J R Soc Med* 74:283, 1981.

Insel TR, Kalin NH, Guttmacher LB, et al: The DST in patients with primary obsessive-compulsive disorder. *Psychiatry Res* 6:153–160, 1982.

Jackson JE, Bressler R: Prescribing tricyclic antidepressant: Part III: Management of overdose. *Drug Therapy* 12(2):175–189, 1982.

Jaffe CM: First-degree atrioventricular block during lithium carbonate treatment. *Am J Psychiatry* 134:88–89, 1977.

Jefferson JW: Lithium and affective disorder in the elderly. *Compr Psychiatry* 24:166–178, 1983.

Jefferson JW, Greist JH: *Primer of Lithium Therapy.* Baltimore, Williams & Wilkins Co, 1977.

Jefferson JW, Marshall JR: *Neuropsychiatric Features of Medical Disorders.* New York, Plenum Press, 1981.

Jenike MA: Dexamethasone suppression: A biological marker of depression. *Drug Therapy.* 12:(9):203–212, 1982a.

Jenike MA: Dexamethasone suppression test as an aid to diagnosing, treating, and following depression in elderly patients. *Topics in Geriatrics* 1:13–15, 1982b.

Jenike MA: ECT and diabetes mellitus. *Am J Psychiatry* 139:136, 1982c.

Jenike MA: Drug treatment of depression. *Topics in Geriatrics* 2:9–11, 1983a.

Jenike MA: Depression in the elderly. *Topics in Geriatrics* 1:33, 1983b.

Jenike MA: Dexamethasone suppression test as a clinical aid in elderly depressed patients. *J Am Geriatr Soc* 31:45–48, 1983c.

Jenike MA: Tardive dyskinesia: Special risk in the elderly. *J Am Geriatr Soc* 31:71–73, 1983d.

Jenike MA: Dyskinesia associated with amoxapine (Ascendin) antidepressant therapy. *Topics in Geriatrics* 1:56, 1983e.

Jenike MA: Alcohol and antihistamines not contraindicated with MAOIs? *Am J Psychiatry* 140:1107, 1983f.

Jenike MA: Treatment of depressed elderly patients with monoamine oxidase inhibitors. *Topics in Geriatrics* 2:13, 1983g.

Jenike MA: Electroconvulsive therapy. *Topics in Geriatrics* 1:37–38, 1983h.

Jenike MA: Depressed in the ER. *Emergency Med* 16:102–120, 1984a.

Jenike MA: The use of monoamine oxidase inhibitors in elderly depressed patients. *J Am Geriatr Soc* 32:571–575, 1984b.

Jenike MA: Electroconvulsive therapy: What are the facts? *Geriatrics* 38:33–38, 1984c.

Jenike MA: MAO inhibitors as treatment for depressed patients with primary degenerative dementia (Alzheimer's disease). *Am J Psychiatry* 1985 (in press).

Jenike MA, Albert MS: The dexamethasone suppression test in patients with presenile and senile dementia of the Alzheimer's type. *J Am Geriatr Soc* 32:441–444, 1984.

Jenike MA, Anderson WH: Depression: Emergency assessment and differential diagnosis, in Manschreck TC, Murray GB (eds): *Psychiatric Medicine Update.* New York, Elsevier, 1984, pp 55–71.

Judd LL, Hubbard B, Janowsky DS, et al: The effect of lithium carbonate on the cognitive functions of normal subjects. *Arch Gen Psychiatry* 34:355–357, 1977.

Jukiz W, Meikle AW, Levinson RA, et al: Effect of diphenylhydantoin on the metabolism of dexamethasone: Mechanism of abnormal dexamethasone suppression in humans. *N Engl J Med* 283:11–14, 1970.

Kalin NH, Risch SC, Janowsky DS, et al: Use of the dexamethasone suppression test in clinical psychiatry. *J Clin Psychopharmacol* 1(2):64–69, 1981.

Kaplitz SE: Withdrawn, apathetic geriatric patients responsive to methylphenidate. *J Am Geriatr Soc* 23:271–276, 1975.

Kayton W, Raskind M: Treatment of depression in the medically ill elderly with methylphenidate. *Am J Psychiatry* 137:963–965, 1980.

Kaufmann MW: Use of methylphenidate in the elderly. *Topics in Geriatrics* 1:3–4, 1982.

Kaufmann MW, Murray GB, Cassem NH: Use of psychostimulants in medically ill depressed patients. *Psychosomatics* 23:817–819, 1982.

Kaufmann MW, Cassem NH, Murray GB, et al: Use of psychostimulants in medically ill patients with neurological disease and major depression. *Can J Psychiatry* 29:46–49, 1984.

Kay DWK, Bergman K: Physical disability and mental health in old age. *J Psychosom Res* 10:3–12, 1966.

Klein DF, Davis JM: *Diagnosis and Drug Treatment of Psychiatric Disorders.* Baltimore, Williams & Wilkins Co, 1969.

Krauthammer C, Klerman GL: Secondary mania. *Arch Gen Psychiatry* 35:1333–1339, 1978.

Krenzelok EP, North DS: Physostigmine's use questioned for amoxapine overdose, letter. *Am J Hosp Pharm* 38:1882–1883, 1981.

Kronfol Z, Greden J, Carroll B: Psychiatric aspects of diabetes mellitus. *Br J Psychiatry* 139:172, 1981.

Kronig MH, Roose SP, Walsh BT, et al: Blood pressure effects of phenelzine. *J Clin Psychopharmacol* 3:307, 1983.

Kulig K, Rumack BH, Sullivan JB: Amoxapine overdose: Coma and seizures without cardiotoxic effects. *JAMA* 248:1092–1094, 1982.

Lapierre YD, Anderson K: Dyskinesia associated with amoxapine antidepressant therapy: A case report. *Am J Psychiatry* 140:493–494, 1983.

Lazare A: Unresolved grief, in Lazare A (ed): *Outpatient Psychiatry.* Baltimore, Williams & Wilkins, 1979, pp 498–512.

Lipsey JR, Pearlson GD, Robinson RG, et al: Nortriptyline treatment of poststroke depression: A double-blind study. *Lancet* 1:297–300, 1984.

Liptzin B: Treatment of mania, in Salzman C (ed): *Clinical Geriatric Psychopharmacology.* New York, McGraw-Hill Book Co, 1984, pp 116–131.

Litovitz TL, Trautman WG: Amoxapine overdose: Seizures and fatalities. *JAMA* 250:1069–1071, 1983.

Louie AK, Meltzer HY: Lithium potentiation of antidepressant treatment. *J Clin Psychopharmacol* 4:316–321, 1984.

Lydiard RB, Gelenberg AJ: Amoxapine: An antidepressant with some neuroleptic properties? *Pharmacotherapy* 1:163–175, 1981.

Maas JW: Biogenic amines and depression. *Arch Gen Psychiatry* 32:1357–1361, 1975.

Makeeva VL, Gol'davskach IL, Pozdnyakova SL: Somatic changes and side effects from the use of lithium salts in the prevention of affective disorders. *Zh Neuropatol Psikhiatr* 74:602–607, 1974.

Martin JB, Reichlin S, Brown GM: Regulation of ACTH secretion and its disorders, in Martin JB, Reichlin S, Brown GM (Eds): *Clinical Neuroendocrinology.* Philadelphia, FA Davis Co, 1977, pp 179–200.

McAllister TW, Ferrell RB, Price TRP, et al: The dexamethasone suppression test in two patients with severe depressive pseudodementia. *Am J Psychiatry* 139(4):479–481, 1982.

McDonald WJ, Golper TA, Mass RD, et al: Adrenocorticotropin-cortisol axis abnormalities in hemodialysis patients. *J Clin Endocrinol Metab* 48:92–97, 1979.

The Medical Letter: Monoamine oxidase inhibitors for depression. July 11, 1980, p 58.

Meyer D, Halfin V: Toxicity secondary to meperidine in patients on monoamine oxidase inhibitors: A case report and critical review. *J Clin Psychopharmacology* 1:319, 1981.

Michael MI, Smith RE, Hermich EM: Adrenal suppression and intranasally applied steroids. *Ann Allergy* 25:569-574, 1967.

Mielke DH: Adverse reactions to thymoleptics, in Gallant DM, Simpson GM (eds): *Depression: Behavioral, Biochemical, Diagnostic and Treatment Concepts*. Holliswood, NY, Spectrum Publications, 1976.

Mitchell RS: Fatal toxic encephalitis occurring during iproniazid therapy and pulmonary tuberculosis. *Ann Intern Med* 42:417, 1955.

Moffie HS, Paykel ES: Depression in medical inpatients. *Br J Psychiatry* 126:346-353, 1975.

Moriarty RW: Tricyclic antidepressant poisoning. *Drug Ther Hosp* 6(8):73-82, 1981.

Murphy JE, Ankier SI: An evaluation of trazodone in the treatment of depression. *Neuropharmacology* 19:1217-1218, 1980.

Myerson A: The effect of benzadrine on fatigue in normal and neurotic persons. *AMA Arch Neurol Psychiatry* 36:816-822, 1936.

Neil JF, Licata SM, May SJ, et al: Dietary noncompliance during treatment with tranylcypromine. *J Clin Psychiatry* 40:33-37, 1979.

Newton R: The side effect profile of trazodone in comparison to an active control and placebo. *J Clin Psychopharmacol* 1(65):895-935, 1981.

Nicotra MB, Rivera M, Pool JL, et al: Tricyclic antidepressant overdose: Clinical and pharmacologic observations. *Clin Toxicol* 18:599-613, 1981.

Normand PS, Jenike MA: Lowered insulin requirements after ECT. *Psychosomatics* 25:418-419, 1984.

Nuller JL, Ostroumova MN: Resistance to inhibiting effect of dexamethasone in patients with endogenous depression. *Acta Psychiatr Scand* 61:169-177, 1980.

Ogura C, Okuma T, Uchida Y, et al: Combined thyroid (triiodothyronine)-tricyclic antidepressant treatment in depressive states. *Folia Psychiatr Neurol Jpn* 28:179-186, 1974.

Orr DA, Bramble MG: Tricyclic antidepressant poisoning and prolonged external cardiac massage during asystole. *Br Med J* 283:1107-1108, 1981.

Oxenkrug GF: Dexamethasone test in alcoholics. *Lancet* 1:794, 1978.

Papp C, Benaim S: Toxic effects of iproniazid in a patient with angina. *Br Med J* 2:1070, 1958.

Pentel P, Sioris L: Incidence of late arrhythmias following tricyclic antidepressant overdose. *Clin Toxicol* 18:543-548, 1981.

Quitkin FM, Rabkin JG, Ross D, et al: Duration of antidepressant drug treatment. *Arch Gen Psychiatry* 41:238-245, 1984.

Raskind M, Peskind E, Rivard MF, et al: DST and cortisol circadian rhythm in primary degenerative dementia. *Am J Psychiatry* 139:1468-1471, 1982.

Rauch PK, Jenike MA: Digoxin toxicity possibly precipitated by trazodone. *Psychosomatics* 25:334-335, 1984.

Rees LH, Besser GM, Jeffcoate WJ, et al: Alcohol induced pseudo-Cushing's syndrome. *Lancet* 1:726, 1977.

Reimann IW, Frolich JC: Effects of diclofenac on lithium kinetics. *Clin Pharmacol Ther* 30:348-352, 1981.

Resnick H, Cantor J: Gerifacts. *Geriatrics* 22:68, 1967.

Richelson E: Pharmacology of antidepressants in use in the United States. *J Clin Psychiatry* 43(11)(sect 2):4–11, 1982.

Robinson DS, Nies A, Revaris CL, et al: Clinical pharmacology of phenelzine. *Arch Gen Psychiatry* 35:629, 1978.

Robinson RG: Depression in aphasic patients: Frequency, severity, and clinicopathological correlations. *Brain Lang* 14:282–291, 1981.

Robinson RG, Szetela B: Mood change following left hemisphere brain injury. *Ann Neurol* 9:447–453, 1981.

Robinson RG, Kubos KL, Starr LB, et al: Mood changes in stroke patients: Relationship to lesion location. *Compr Psychiatry* 24:555–566, 1983.

Roth M: The natural history of mental disorder in old age. *J Ment Sci* 101:281–301, 1955.

Rowe JW, Andres R, Tobin JD, et al: The effect of age on creatinine clearance in men: A cross-sectional and longitudinal study. *J Gerontol* 31:155–163, 1976.

Rudorfer MV, Clayton PJ: Depression, dementia, and dexamethasone suppression, letter. *Am J Psychiatry* 138:701, 1981.

Rudorfer MV, Young RC: Desipramine: Cardiovascular effects and plasma levels. *Am J Psychiatry* 137:984–986, 1980.

Sachar EJ, Asnis G, Halbreich U, et al: Recent studies in the neuroendocrinology of major depressive disorders. *Psychiatr Clin North Am* 3:313–326, 1980.

Sachar EJ, Halbreich U, Asnis GM, et al: Paradoxical cortisol responses to dextroamphetamine in endogenous depression. *Arch Gen Psychiatry* 38:1113–1117, 1981.

Sachar EJ, Hellman L, Roffwarg HP, et al: Disrupted 24-hour patterns of cortisol secretion in psychotic depression. *Arch Gen Psychiatry* 28:19–24, 1973.

Salzman C: A primer on geriatric psychopharmacology. *Am J Psychiatry* 139:67–76, 1982.

Schlesser MA, Winokur G, Sherman BM: Hypothalamic-pituitary-adrenal axis activity in depressive illness: Its relationship to classification. *Arch Gen Psychiatry* 37:737–743, 1980.

Scovern AW, Kilmann PR: Status of ECT: A review of the outcome literature. *Psychol Bull* 87:260, 1980.

Sendbuehler J, Goldstein S: Attempted suicide among the aged. *J Am Geriatr Soc* 25:245–248, 1977.

Sheehan DV, Claycomb JB, Kouretas N: Monoamine oxidase inhibitors: prescription and patient management. *Int J Psychiatry Med* 10:99, 1980–1981.

Silberman EK: Heterogeneity of amphetamine response in depressed patients. *Am J Psychiatry* 138:1302–1306, 1981.

Smith SR, Biedsoe T, Chetii MK: Cortisol metabolism and the pituitary-adrenal axis in adults with protein-calorie malnutrition. *J Clin Endocrinol Metab* 40:43–52, 1975.

Snyder SH, Yamamura HI: Antidepressants and the muscarinic acetylcholine receptor. *Arch Gen Psychiatry* 34:236–239, 1977.

Spar JE, Gerner R: Does the dexamethasone suppression test distinguish dementia from depression? *Am J Psychiatry* 139:238–240, 1982.

Spar JE, LaRue A: Major depression in the elderly: DSM III criteria and the dexamethasone suppression test as predictors of treatment response. *Am J Psychiatry* 140:844–847, 1983.

Streeten DHP, Stevenson CT, Dalakos TC, et al: The diagnosis of hypercortisolism, biochemical criteria differentiating patients from lean and obese normal subjects and from females on oral contraceptives. *J Clin Endocrinol Metab* 29:119–121, 1969.

Task Force on the use of Laboratory tests in psychiatry: tricyclic antidepressants — blood level measurements and clinical outcome. *AM J Psychiatry* 142:142–149, 1985.

Tollefson GD, Senogles SE, Frey II WH, et al: A comparison of peripheral and central human muscarinic cholinergic receptor affinities for psychotropic drugs. *Biol Psychiatry* 5:555–567, 1982.

Tourigny-Rivard MF, Raskind M, Rivard D: The dexamethasone suppression test in an elderly population. *Biol Psychiatry* 16:1177–1184, 1981.

Tsuang MT, Woolson RF, Fleming JA: Premature deaths in schizophrenia and affective disorders. *Arch Gen Psychiatry* 37:979–983, 1980.

Tsutsui S, Yamazaki Y, Namba T, et al: Combined therapy of T and antidepressants in depression. *J Int Med Res* 7:138–146, 1979.

Veith RC, Raskind MA, Caldwell JH, et al: Cardiovascular effects of tricyclic antidepressants. *N Engl J Med* 306:954–959, 1982.

Wallace EZ, Rosmann P, Toshav N, et al: Pituitary-adrenocorticol function in chronic renal failure: Studies in episodic secretion of cortisol and dexamethasone suppressability. *J Clin Endocrinol Metab* 50:46–51, 1980.

Weiner RD: The role of electroconvulsive therapy in the treatment of depression in the elderly. *J Am Geriatr Soc* 30:710–712, 1982.

Wellens H, Cats B, Durren D: Symptomatic sinus node abnormalities following lithium carbonate therapy. *Am J Med* 59:285–287, 1975.

Wells BG, Gelenberg AJ: Chemistry, pharmacology, pharmacokinetics, adverse effects and efficacy of the antidepressant maprotiline hydrochloride. *Pharmacotherapy* 1:121–139, 1981.

Wells CE: Pseudodementia. *Am J Psychiatry* 136:895–900, 1979.

Wells CE: Pseudodementia. *Am J Psychiatry* 120:244–249, 1963.

White K, MacDonald N, Razini J, et al: *Compr Psychiatry* 24:453–457, 1983.

Wilson J, Kraus E, Bailas M, et al: Reversible sinus node abnormalities due to lithium carbonate therapy. *N Engl J Med* 294:1223–1224, 1976.

Wolf PA, Dawber TR, Thomas HE, et al: Epidemiology of stroke, in Thompson RA, Green JR (eds): *Advances in Neurology*. New York, Raven Press, 1977, pp 5–19.

Zavodnick S: Atrial flutter with amoxapine: A case report. *Am J Psychiatry* 138:1503–1504, 1981.

"Aging is when you have too much room in the house and not enough room in the medicine cabinet."

CHAPTER 5

Anxiety

Anxiety is a universal human experience and generally should not be regarded as an indication for medication. It can, however, reach disabling proportions and can also be associated with phobias and panic attacks. Numerous factors, such as loss of friends and loved ones, failing health, intellectual decline, feelings of helplessness and worthlessness, and loss of control over their immediate environment, make the elderly particularly susceptible to anxiety states. Even though roughly 11% of the population is over age 65, this groups uses about 25% of all prescription and over-the-counter drugs sold, a large proportion of which are aimed at the alleviation of anxiety. For these reasons, physicians who care for the elderly should be aware of a number of special considerations that apply when prescribing antianxiety drugs for these patients (Jenike 1982a; 1983a; Altesman and Cole, 1983).

DIFFERENTIAL DIAGNOSIS

Before beginning pharmacologic treatment, it is important to rule out medical causes of anxiety (Table 5-1) and to discuss with the patient possible precipitating factors. Occasionally, treatment of a medical condition will resolve superimposed anxious feelings. For example, the patient with hypoxia secondary to congestive heart failure may feel much less anxious after treatment with digitalis and a diuretic (Dietch, 1981).

When there is a clear precipitating event, discussion of the problem or suggestion of an alternate solution may be adequate. If an elderly person in a nursing home is anxious, for example, because the patient in the next bed died last evening, it would be inappropriate to treat such anxiety initially with medication. Occasionally, the anxiety can be alleviated by environmental manipulation or by discussing the

Table 5-1
Medical Causes of Anxiety

Cardiovascular	*Endocrinologic* (continued)
Myocardial infarction	Carcinoid syndrome
Paroxysmal atrial tachycardia	Hypothermia
Mitral valve prolapse	Cushing's disease
	Hyperkalemia
Dietary	
Caffeine	*Hematologic*
Vitamin deficiencies	Anemia
Drug-Related	*Immunologic*
Akathisia	Systemic lupus erythematosus
Anticholinergic toxicity	
Antihypertensive side effects	*Neurologic*
Digitalis toxicity	CNS infections
Withdrawal syndromes: alcohol,	CNS masses
sedative-hypnotics	Toxins
	Temporal lobe epilepsy
Endocrinologic	Postconcussion syndrome
Insulinoma	
Hypoglycemia	*Pulmonary*
Hypo- or hyperthyroidism	Chronic obstructive lung disease
Hypo- or hypercalcemia	Pneumonia
Pheochromocytoma	Hypoxia

patient's problems in a direct manner. When medical causes have been ruled out and when no precipitating factor for the anxiety can be identified, antianxiety drugs may be useful.

CONSEQUENCES OF ALTERED PHYSIOLOGY IN THE ELDERLY

The clinically significant physiologic concomitants of aging, as reviewed in chapter 2, must be considered before antianxiety agents are prescribed. These include changes in absorption, distribution, protein binding, hepatic metabolism, and renal excretion of drugs. Some of these changes, as they pertain to antianxiety agents, will be briefly reviewed.

There are several age-related changes that may alter drug absorption in the gut of the elderly. Gastric pH increases with age, and this may alter the solubility and absorption of many drugs. Splanchnic blood flow decreases in the elderly. Finally, both active absorption processes and passive transport, which is important in drug absorption, are impaired in the elderly (Omslander, 1981).

The proportion of total body fat may increase from 10% of body weight at age 20 to 24% at age 60. This increases the volume of distribution of lipid soluble drugs, such as diazepam (Valium), and greatly prolongs drug half-life. In addition, body water may decrease from 25% to 18% in the same period. Thus, water-soluble drugs, such as ethanol, will have higher concentrations in the elderly due to an apparent decrease in the size of their reservoir (Crook and Cohen, 1981).

A number of studies have demonstrated a 15% to 25% reduction in serum albumin levels in patients over 60 years of age, as compared with levels in persons under the age of 40 (Schumacher, 1980; Bender et al, 1975; Hayes et al, 1975; Wallace et al, 1976; Greenblatt, 1979). Since most sedatives are highly protein-bound, this decrease in protein-binding sites in the elderly liberates more free active drug into the circulation and increases the risk of toxicity. The activity of hepatic cytochrome P-450 may decrease with age, and demethylation slows, leading to higher levels of unmetabolized drug. After age 40, the glomerular filtration rate (GFR) and renal plasma flow decline progressively, to approximately 50% of normal by age 70 (Papper, 1978). This results in a longer duration of drug action, and increases the likelihood of toxicity if dosage is not adjusted.

In addition to these pharmacokinetic changes in the elderly, decreased CNS dopamine and acetylcholine levels can lead to increased sensitivity to extrapyramidal and anticholinergic side effects, respectively. An increased tendency to CNS disinhibition increases the likelihood of drug-associated confusion, sedation, and paradoxical reactions.

EARLY ANTIANXIETY AGENTS

In the early twentieth century, bromides were used as antianxiety drugs. In the 1930s, however, they were implicated as the cause of a toxic delirium, which resulted from their accumulation with chronic use. Until the early 1950s, phenobarbital was also commonly used as an antianxiety agent, and shorter-acting barbiturates such as secobarbital and amobarbital were used as hypnotics. However, the potential for tolerance, physical dependence, and the development of a life-threatening withdrawal syndrome with these drugs made them far from ideal.

After meprobamate (Miltown) was introduced, it became so popular that manufacturers could not keep up with the demand, even though it differed only slightly from barbiturates (Hollister, 1978). The structure of meprobamate was manipulated to produce numerous similar drugs such as glutethimide and methyprylon (Noludar). As dissatisfaction with the barbiturates increased, other drugs, such as ethchlorvynol (Placidyl), enjoyed a brief period of popularity. The enthusiasm for these drugs dwindled, however, as clinicians realized that they had many of the same drawbacks as the barbiturates. Meprobamate, for example, carries an unacceptable risk of addiction and fatality on overdose. In fact, the addicting dose overlaps with the therapeutic range. Although the therapeutic range is 1200 to 2400 mg/d (Baldessarini, 1977), physical signs of withdrawal can occur with the discontinuation of doses as low as 1200 mg/d; severe withdrawal signs and seizures can be expected at doses above 3200 mg/d.

Although these drugs are still on the market, with the advent of safer and more effective medications, such as the benzodiazepines, they no longer have a place in the treatment of anxiety in the elderly.

BENZODIAZEPINES

Introduced in 1960, chlordiazepoxide was the first benzodiazepine to come on the market. Many others soon followed, including diazepam, flurazepam (Dalmane), clorazepate dipotassium (Tranxene), oxazepam (Serax), lorazepam (Ativan), and prazepam (Centrax). The benzodiazepines have been shown to be superior to placebo, barbiturates, meprobamate, and the sedative-type antihistamines in most clinical trials of anxious patients (Cole, 1978; Davies et al, 1977; Douglas 1975, Bernstein, 1979; Salzman, 1981), although no one benzodiazepine has been shown to be superior to any other in relieving anxiety.

In the elderly, benzodiazepines are closer to the ideal sedative-hypnotic than other drugs currently available. They are less addicting than the antianxiety drugs typically used in earlier years, and are unlikely to cause lethal overdosage when taken alone. Most of the fatalities associated with benzodiazepine overdosage have occurred when other respiratory depressants, such as alcohol, were also ingested.

Each of the benzodiazepines produces more sedation as dosage is increased, but antianxiety effects are exhibited at lower doses. This has been attributed to their primary action on the limbic system, which is believed to control anxiety, fear, and rage. Since no benzodiazepine has been shown to be better at relieving anxiety than any other (Baldessarini, 1977; Cole, 1978; Davies et al, 1977; Douglas, 1975), the choice of individual drugs for the elderly should be based on the potential for serious side effects.

Although there are many similarities among the benzodiazepines,

Table 5-2
Comparison of Benzodiazepine Anxiolytics

Drug	Rate of Onset	Half-Life (h)	Active Metabolites	Half-Life of Metabolites (h)	Doses (mg/d) Adult	Doses (mg/d) Elderly	Route of Administration
Oxazepam (Serax)	Intermediate to slow	5–15	None	–	10–60	10–30	Oral
Lorazepam (Ativan)	Intermediate	10–20	None	–	1–4	0.5–4.0	Oral, IM, IV
Diazepam (Valium)	Fastest	26–53	Yes	36–200	5–30	2–10	Oral, IM, IV†
Chlordiazepoxide HCl (Librium)	Intermediate	8–28	Yes	36–200	10–100	5–30	Oral, IM, IV†
Prazepam (Centrax)	Slow	30–200	Yes	36–200	20–60	10–15	Oral
Clorazepate dipotassium (Tranxene)	Fast	30–200	Yes	36–200	15–60	7.5–15	Oral
Alprazolam (Xanax)	Intermediate	6–15	Yes	*	0.25–2.0	0.125–0.5	Oral
Halazepam (Paxipam)	Intermediate to slow	14	Yes	36–200	20–120		Oral
Triazolam (Halcion)	Fast	2–5	–	–	0.25–0.5	0.25–0.5	Oral
Temazepam (Restoril)	Intermediate to slow	12–24	–	–	15–30	15–30	Oral

*Unknown; probably about the same as the parent drug.
†IM doses unreliably absorbed.

there are interdrug differences that are clinically significant in elderly patients (Table 5-2). Benzodiazepines can be divided into two groups on the basis of metabolism.

Short-Acting Agents

The first group consists of relatively short-acting drugs that are simply conjugated to glucuronide in the liver and then eliminated in the urine (Greenblatt, 1980). Lorazepam and oxazepam, the two drugs in this category, are especially attractive choices for use in the elderly because they have a short half-life, have no active metabolites, and their metabolism is affected only slightly, if at all, by the physiologic changes that accompany aging. The main disadvantage of these drugs is that they may have to be given more than once a day. Initial dosage should be 10 mg of exazepam or 0.5 mg of lorazepam two or three times daily. Lorazepam is the only benzodiazepine that is well absorbed intramuscularly (Schuckit, 1983; 1984) and may be particularly useful when oral dosing is impossible.

Long-Acting Agents

Drugs in the second category, such as diazepam, chlordiazepoxide, clorazepate, and prazepam, have a long duration of action, have active metabolites, and are slowly eliminated from the body. Their metabolism is profoundly affected by the physiologic concomitants of aging. For example, the half-life of diazepam, which is 20 hours at age 20, increases to 90 hours at age 80 (Rosenbaum, 1979). The long half-lives of these drugs in the elderly can lead to accumulation with deleterious clinical effects. Their advantage, however, is that they can be given once a day or even every other day. Initial dosages of these drugs should be in the range of 2 to 5 mg/day of diazepam or its equivalent. Dosage should be increased cautiously, because it may take more than a week for steady-state levels to be reached with the longer-acting drugs.

Alprazolam (Xanax) is a new benzodiazepine which is metabolized extensively in the liver. A number of metabolites have been identified but, because of their rapid clearance, none is known to exert significant biologic action (Abernathy et al, 1983a). The elimination half-life of alprazolam increases significantly with advancing age in men but not in women. The mean half-life in young males is 11 hours and this increases to 19 hours in elderly males (Greenblatt et al, 1983).

Benzodiazepine Withdrawal

The physical manifestations of withdrawal syndromes due to abrupt discontinuation of any of the benzodiazepines are similar (Jenike, 1984). However, drugs with longer half-lives tend to produce onset of withdrawal syndromes later than those with shorter half-lives (Hollister, 1961; Pevnick et al, 1978; Einarson, 1980; Khan, 1980; Jenike, 1984). Minor withdrawal symptoms include eleveated pulse and respiration rates, postural hypotension, coarse rhythmic intention tremors, hyperreflexia, muscular weakness and aching, apprehension, anorexia, insomnia, and profuse sweating. Severe withdrawal symptoms may include hyperthermia, delirium, generalized convulsions, and psychosis. Psychosis is characterized by paranoia with visual and auditory hallucinations.

Because withdrawal seizures are thought to be due to a rapid drop in blood level, patients who have been on large doses for a long time should be very slowly tapered off the drug. Addicting doses of diazepam have been estimated at 80 to 120 mg for 40 to 50 days; for chlordiazepoxide, 300 to 600 mg for 60 to 180 days (Jenike, 1984). Addicting doses of the shorter-acting agents are more difficult to estimate, but there is one report of a patient who took 12 mg of lorazepam daily who had a grand mal seizure 72 hours after stopping the drug (Einarson, 1980).

Memory Impairment with Benzodiazepines

There are a number of anecdotal reports that various benzodiazepines can interfere with memory (Angus and Romney, 1984; Scharf et al, 1983; Pandit et al, 1976; Bixler et al, 1979; Roth et al, 1980; McKay and Dundee, 1980; Petersen and Ghoneim, 1980; Barclay, 1982; George and Dundee, 1977; Kothary et al, 1981). Some authors feel that benzodiazepines interfere with both short-term and long term memory, and most feel that they interfere with the memory consolidation process.

On the other hand, some investigators have found that benzodiazepines actually enhance recall (Brown et al, 1978; Liljequist, 1978; Hartley, 1980) and others found that in a sample of normal student volunteers that a low dose of diazepam (5 mg) impaired the short-term memory of low-anxiety subjects but actually improved the memory of high anxiety subjects (Barnett et al, 1981).

Clinically, one does not frequently see isolated memory deficits in elderly patients who are not oversedated.

Benzodiazepines in Patients with Liver Disease

Since the benzodiazepines are metabolized by the liver, special considerations apply when using these agents in patients with hepatic disease. Cirrhosis produces a two- to threefold increase in the half-life of both diazepam and chlordiazepoxide relative to age-matched controls (Wilkinson and Schenker, 1975; 1976; Klotz et al, 1975; Ochs et al, 1983). The predominant cause of this is a significant reduction in plasma clearance but the distribution of the drugs is also slightly increased due to a reduction in plasma binding. Acute viral hepatitis has a similar but slightly smaller effect upon plasma clearance, which is reversable upon clinical recovery. Neither of these diseases has a significant effect on the disposition of oxazepam and lorazepam (Wilkinson and Schenker, 1975; 1976).

Ochs and colleagues clearly demonstrated that cirrhotic patients developed more self-rated daytime sedation than normal controls when given diazepam. Sedation strongly correlated with total levels of diazepam and its major metabolite desmethyldiazepam (Ochs et al, 1983). They concluded that reduced hepatic clearance of diazepam in cirrhotics leads to increased accumulation during long-term dosing and they recommended that diazepam could probably be given to cirrhotics safely provided daily dosage is reduced by approximately 50%.

In elderly patients with liver disease, it is probably wisest to use lorazepam or oxazepam since we know that their metabolism is not significantly altered by such disease.

Benzodiazepines in Patients with Lung Disease

In general, benzodiazepines are felt to be safer drugs than barbiturates in terms of respiratory depression associated with overdosage (Cohn, 1983). A number of studies have shown that the longer-acting benzodiazepines do, in fact, have significant respiratory depressant effects (Utting and Pleuvry, 1975; Cohn, 1983; Rao et al, 1973; Huch and Huch, 1974; Catchlove and Kafer, 1971; Kronenberg et al, 1975). In contrast, the short-acting agents seem to be much less likely to depress respiration. Steen et al (1966) gave intravenous (IV) oxazepam (only approved for oral use) to four volunteers and could show no statistically significant change in the response to breathing elevated carbon dioxide levels. Others have reported actual respiratory stimulation after oral doses of lorazepam (Dodson et al, 1976) and triazolam (Elliott et al, 1975). Temazepam in oral doses of 40 mg, but not 20 mg, significantly depressed the ventilatory response to carbon dioxide in 12 healthy volunteers (Pleuvry et al, 1980).

Denaut and colleagues (1975) compared the respiratory effects of lorazepam and diazepam in 20 patients with chronic obstructive lung disease. Both drugs induced a respiratory depression with slight respiratory acidosis, but lorazepam caused no significant hypoxemia. They concluded that the respiratory depressant effects of both lorazepam and diazepam are modest; nevertheless, preference should be given to lorazepam because of its less prolonged duration of action with no modification of the PaO_2. At the present time, the bulk of the data support lorazepam as the drug of first choice in the anxious elderly patient with significant lung disease.

OTHER ANTIANXIETY AGENTS

Other drugs which have been used to treat anxiety are listed in Table 5-3.

Antihistamines

Antihistamines such as diphenhydramine (Benadryl) and hydroxyzine (Atarax, Vistaril) are sometimes prescribed for anxiety or insomnia,

Table 5-3
Nonbenzodiazepine Anxiolytics

Type	Representative Drugs	Dose (mg)	Side-effects
Antihistamines	Diphenhydramine	25	Anticholinergic
	Hydroxyzine	25	Sedation
Neuroleptics*	*High-potency*		
	Haloperidol	0.5 bid	Extrapyramidal Dystonia
	Thiothixene	1 bid	Akathesia
	Fluphenazine	1 bid	Tardive dyskinesia
	Low-potency		
	Chlorpromazine	10 bid	Orthostatic hypotension
	Thioridazine	10 bid	Sedation
			Tardive dyskinesia
β-Blockers	Propranolol	40 qid†	Contraindications
	Atenolol	50–100	Asthma
			Sinus bradycardia
			Congestive heart failure

*See chapter 3.
†Kathol et al (1980).

and they are also common ingredients in over-the-counter agents. Although frequently effective, antihistamines have many potential side effects, including disturbed coordination, weakness, inability to concentrate, urinary frequency, palpitations, and hypotension. In addition, their anticholinergic properties make them poor choices for patients taking other anticholinergic agents, such as tricyclic antidepressants, neuroleptics, and antiarrhythmic agents. An acute toxic delirium may result when antihistamines are coadministered with these agents, with such classic anticholinergic signs as blurred vision, dryness of the mouth, urinary retention, tachycardia, and constipation.

Antihistamines may be most useful in elderly patients with severe chronic obstructive lung disease (COLD), whose respiration may be easily depressed by other antianxiety agents. Antihistamines are much less likely to depress respiratory drive than most other drugs, except perhaps the high-potency neuroleptics. In patients with severe lung disease, sedatives could worsen respiratory depression and thereby, paradoxically, increase anxiety. If increasing anxiety is treated by an increase in medication, a lethal spiral may result (Shader and Greenblatt, 1977).

Neuroleptics

Neuroleptics are sometimes used in the treatment of severe anxiety and agitation. Low doses of a high-potency neuroleptic, such as haloperidol (Haldol), thiothixene (Navane), or fluphenazine (Permitil, Prolixin), are preferred in the elderly. Low-potency neuroleptics, such as chlorpromazine (Thorazine) and thioridazine (Mellaril), have more associated hypotensive, cardiovascular, and anticholinergic side effects. The low-potency agents may be preferred in patients suffering from movement disorders such as Parkinson's disease where they will be less likely to exacerbate extrapyramidal symptoms (see chapter 3). Patients with organic brain disease may feel much better and exhibit less agitation, paranoia, antisocial behavior, and insomnia with doses as low as 0.5 mg of haloperidol (Haldol) or 1 mg of thiothixene (Navane) twice daily. Chlorpromazine and thioridazine should be used with initial doses as low as 10 mg twice daily (Jenike, 1985).

Neuroleptics should be used with caution, because the data are now fairly conclusive that elderly patients are much more sensitive to side effects such as tardive dyskinesia (Jenike, 1983b) (see chapter 3).

β-Blockers

Since anxiety often has both psychological and somatic components—palpitations, diaphoresis, tremulousness, urinary frequency, and tachycardia, which are mediated by the sympathetic nervous system—it is occasionally recommended that β-blockers be used to alleviate this type of anxiety (Omslander, 1981; James, 1909; Pitts and McClure, 1967). Some investigators even believe that sometimes anxiety is the subjective feeling resulting primarily from the somatic manifestations (James, 1909); that is, one feels anxious because his or her heart beats fast, rather than the tachycardia being a result of the anxiety. Others have reproduced panic attacks by infusing lactate into susceptible patients (Pitts and McClure, 1967).

Agents such as propranolol hydrochloride (Inderal) can be used to block the peripheral sympathetic concomitants of anxiety. One study (Kathol et al, 1980) reported that propranolol, 40 mg four times daily, not only reduced the somatic concomitants of anxiety, but also improved the psychological symptoms, such as apprehension and irritability. Propranolol may be helpful in patients who have clear-cut somatic concomitants to anxiety. Contraindications such as asthma, sinus bradycardia, and heart failure must be heeded.

Antidepressants

The depressed patient who is also anxious may respond best to low doses of a tricyclic antidepressant or, in more extreme cases, to electroconvulsive therapy. In fact, antianxiety drugs alone may make the depressed patient feel worse. Many depressed elderly patients show such classic signs of depression as decreased appetite and sleeplessness (or increased appetite and somnolence), inability to concentrate, fatigue, guilt, suicidal ideation, and psychomotor retardation or agitation. Some patients, however, appear more demented than depressed. A rapidly progressive dementia, especially in a previously depressed elderly patient, should alert the clinician to the possibility of pseudodementia secondary to depression (Wells, 1979; Jenike, 1982a).

Antidepressant drugs should never be used to treat primary anxiety, because they are not as efficacious as the benzodiazepines, they have a considerably greater potential for side effects, and they are extremely dangerous if taken in overdose.

DRUG INTERACTIONS

Since elderly patients frequently suffer medical problems, they often take several medications concomitantly. Among the drugs commonly used in the elderly that have CNS depressant effects are antihypertensive medications (methyldopa, reserpine, or clonidine), other sedative-hypnotics, analgesics, tricyclic antidepressants, MAOIs, and neuroleptics. It is therefore crucial to remember that, when combined with antianxiety medication, these CNS depressant effects are additive. Such effects may be manifested by a variety of symptoms, including dysarthria, diplopia, ataxia, blurred vision, confusion, dizziness, vertigo, nystagmus, muscle weakness, lack of coordination, and somnolence (Shader and Greenblatt, 1977; Byck, 1975). Patients with underlying organic brain disease are more prone to such effects from benzodiazepines alone, or in combination with other drugs.

Blood levels of most of the benzodiazepines (including alprazolam) are increased by more than one third when cimetidine is used concomitantly (Klotz and Reimann 1980a; Desmond et al, 1980; Abernathy et al, 1983b; Klotz and Reimann, 1980b). With the rapid increase in cimetidine use, it is important to keep this drug interaction in mind. Cimetidine does not, however, interfere with the metabolism of the short-acting benzodiazepines, such as lorazepam and oxazepam, which are eliminated exclusively after conjugation as glucuronide (Patwardhan et al, 1980; Jenike, 1982b).

TREATMENT GUIDELINES

The following guidelines are suggested for the rational use of antianxiety medications in the elderly:

- Look for a clear-cut precipitating factor for the anxiety, and consider possible organic causes of anxiety.
- Before prescribing medication, try to alleviate the anxiety by manipulating environmental factors or discussing the patient's problems.
- Use benzodiazepines as first-line drugs. Lorazepam and oxazepam are the safest benzodiazepines to use in the elderly, because of their relatively short half-lives and because their metabolism is not altered appreciably by aging or by the concomitant use of other drugs.
- If longer-acting benzodiazepines, such as diazepam, chlordiazepoxide, or prazepam, are chosen, use very low doses once daily or even

every other day. More than a week of therapy will be required to reach a steady state, so increase doses cautiously.

- Abrupt stopping of long-term benzodiazepine usage may precipitate a withdrawal syndrome. Discontinue such usage gradually.
- Oxazepam and lorazepam are probably safest in patients with liver disease. Lorazepam seems the best drug for patients with severe lung disease.
- Antihistamines may be useful in patients with severe chronic obstructive lung disease. Be aware of their anticholinergic side effects.
- Neuroleptics are most useful in severely anxious, agitated, or psychotic patients. Low doses of high-potency neuroleptics are preferred unless patients have a preexisting movement disorder.
- β-blockers, such as propranolol, may occasionally be helpful when anxiety is accompanied by signs of sympathetic overstimulation. Be aware of contraindications to these agents.
- Antidepressants may be useful if the patient is clinically depressed or pseudodemented. They are not as effective as benzodiazepines in treating primary anxiety and are much more dangerous in elderly patients.
- If anxiety persists despite adequate treatment, reevaluate the patient for possible organic causes.

REFERENCES

Abernathy DR, Greenblatt DJ, Divoll M, et al: Pharmacokinetics of alprazolam. *J Clin Psychiatry* 44:45–47, 1983a.

Abernathy DR, Greenblatt DJ, Divoll M, et al: Differential effects of cimetidine on drug oxidation vs. conjugation. *J Pharmacol Exp Ther* 224:508–513, 1983b.

Altesman RI, Cole JO: Psychopharmacologic treatment of anxiety. *J Clin Psychiatry* 44:12–18, 1983.

Angus WR, Romney DM: The effect of diazepam on patients' memory. *J Clin Psychopharmacol* 4:203–206, 1984.

Baldessarini RJ: *Chemotherapy in Psychiatry*. Cambridge, Mass, Harvard University Press, 1977.

Barclay J: Variations in amnesia with intravenous diazepam. *Oral Surg* 53:329–334, 1982.

Barnett DB, Taylor-Davies A, Desai H: Differential effect of diazepam on short-term memory in subjects with high or low level anxiety. *Br J Clin Pharmacol* 11:411–412, 1981.

Bender AD, Post A, Meier JP, et al: Plasma protein binding of drugs as a function of age in adult human subjects. *J Pharm Sci* 64:1711–1713, 1975.

Bernstein JG: Psychotropic drugs in the elderly, in Manschreck T (ed):

Psychiatric Medicine Update. New York, Elsevier-North Holland, 1979, pp 75-89.

Bixler EO, Scharf MB, Soldatos CR, et al: Effects of hypnotic drugs on memory. *Life Sci* 25:1379-1388, 1979.

Brown J, Lewis V, Brown M, et al: Amnesic effects of intravenous diazepam and lorazepam. *Experientia* 34:501-502, 1978.

Byck R: Drugs and the treatment of psychiatric disorders, in Goodman LS, Gilman A (eds): *The Pharmacological Basis of Therapeutics*. New York, Macmillan, 1975, pp 152-200.

Catchlove RFH, Kafer ER: The effects of diazepam on respiration in patients with obstructive pulmonary disease. *Anesthesiology* 34:14-18, 1971.

Cohn MA: Hypnotics and the control of breathing: A review. *Br J Clin Pharmacol* 16:2455-2505, 1983.

Cole JD: Clinical use of antianxiety drugs, in Bernstein JD (ed): *Clinical Psychopharmacology*. Littleton, Mass, PSG Publishing Co, Inc, 1978 14-26.

Crook T, Cohen G (eds): *Physician's Handbook on Psychotherapeutic Drug Use in the Aged*. New Canaan, Conn, Mark Powley Associates, Inc, 1981.

Davies B, et al: Effects on the heart of different tricyclic antidepressants, in Medela J (ed): *Sineguan (Doxepin HCl): A Monograph of Recent Clinical Studies*. Princeton, NJ, Excerpta Medica, 1977, pp 54-58.

Denaut M, Yernault JC, DeCoster A: Double-blind comparison of the respiratory effects of parenteral lorazepam and diazepam in patients with chronic obstructive lung disease. *Curr Med Res Opin* 2:611-615, 1975.

Desmond PV, Patwardhen RV, Schenker S, et al: Cimetidine impairs elimination of chlordiazepoxide in man. *Ann Intern Med* 93:266-268, 1980.

Dietch JT: Diagnosis of organic anxiety disorders. *Psychosomatics* 22:661-669, 1981.

Dodson ME, Yousseff Y, Maddison S, et al: Respiratory effects of lorazepam. *Br J Anaesth* 48:611-612, 1976.

Douglas WW: Histamine and antihistamines: 5-hydroxytryptamine and antagonists, in Goodman LS, Gilman A (eds): *The Pharmacological Basis of Therapeutics*. New York, Macmillan, 1975, pp 590-629.

Einarson TR: Lorazepam withdrawal seizures. *Lancet* 1:151, 1980.

Elliott HW, Navarro G, Kokka N, et al: Early phase I evaluation of sedatives hypnotics or minor tranquilizers, in *Hypnotics, Methods of Development and Evaluation*. New York, Spectrum Publications, 1975, pp 87-108.

George K, Dundee J: Relative amnesic actions of diazepam, flunitrazepam and lorazepam in man. *Br J Psychopharmacol* 4:45-50, 1977.

Greenblatt DJ: Reduced serum albumin concentration in the elderly: A report from the Boston Collaborative Drug Surveillance Program. *J Am Geriatr Soc* 27:20-22, 1979.

Greenblatt DJ: Pharmacokinetic comparisons. Benzodiazepines 1980: Current Update. *Psychosomatics* 21(10)(suppl):9-14, 1980.

Greenblatt DJ, Divoll M, Abernathy DR, et al: Alprazolam kinetics in the elderly: Relation to antipyrine disposition. *Arch Gen Psychiatry* 40:287-290, 1983.

Hartley L: Diazepam: Human learning of different material. *Prog Neuropsychopharmacol* 4:193-197, 1980.

Hayes MJ, et al: Changes in drug metabolism with increasing age: Phenytoin clearance and protein binding. *Br J Clin Pharmacol* 2:73-79, 1975.

Hollister LE: *Clinical Pharmacology of Psychotherapeutic Drugs.* New York, Churchill Livingston, 1978.

Hollister LE, Motzenbecker FP, Degan FO: Withdrawal reactions from chlordiazepoxide. *Pharmacologia* 2:63–68, 1961.

Huch R, Huch A: Respiratory depression after tranquilizers. *Lancet* 1:1267, 1974.

James W: *Psychology.* New York, Holt, 1909.

Jenike MA: Using sedative drugs in the elderly. *Drug Therapy* 12:186–190, 1982a.

Jenike MA: Cimetidine in elderly patients: Review of uses and risks. *J Am Geriatr Soc* 30:170–173, 1982b.

Jenike MA: Treatment of anxiety in elderly patients. *Geriatrics* 38:115–120, 1983a.

Jenike MA: Tardive dyskinesia: Special risk in the elderly. *J Am Geriatr Soc* 31:71–73, 1983b.

Jenike MA: Drug abuse. *Sci Am Med* 7:1–8, 1984.

Jenike MA: Use of psychopharmacologic agents in the elderly, in Goroll AH, May L, Mulley A (eds): *Primary Care Medicine.* Philadelphia, Pa, JB Lippincott Co, 1985.

Kathol RG, et al: Propranolol in chronic anxiety disorders. *Arch Gen Psychiatry* 37:1361–1365, 1980.

Khan A, Joyce P, Jones AV: Benzodiazepine withdrawal syndromes. *NZ Med J* Aug 13, 92:94–96, 1980.

Klotz U, Avant GR, Hoyumpa A, et al: The effects of age and liver disease on the disposition and elimination of diazepam in man. *J Clin Invest* 55:347–359, 1975.

Klotz U, Reimann I: Delayed clearance of diazepam due to cimetidine. *N Engl J Med* 302:1012–1014, 1980a.

Klotz U, Reimann I: Influence of cimetidine on the pharmacokinetics of dismethyldiazepam and oxazepam. *Eur J Clin Pharmacol* 18:517–520, 1980b.

Kothary S, Braun A, Pandit U, et al: Time course of antirecall effect of diazepam and lorazepam following oral administration. *Anesthesiology* 55:641–644, 1981.

Kronenberg RS, Cosio MG, Stevenson JE, et al: The use of oral diazepam in patients with obstructive lung disease and hypercapnia. *Ann Intern Med* 83:83–84, 1975.

Liljequist R, Linnoila M, Mattila M: Effect of diazepam and chlorpromazine on memory functions in man. *Eur J Clin Pharmacol* 13:339–343, 1978.

McKay AC, Dundee JV: Effect of oral benzodiazepines on memory. *Br J Anaesth* 52:1247–1257, 1980.

Ochs HR, Greenblatt DJ, Eckardt B, et al: Repeated diazepam dosing in cirrhotic patients: Cumulation and sedation. *Clin Pharmacol Ther* 33:471–476, 1983.

Omslamder JG: Drug therapy in the elderly. *Ann Intern Med* 94:711–722, 1981.

Pandit SK, Heisterkamp DV, Cohen PJ: Further studies of the antirecall effect of lorazepam. *Anesthesiology* 45:495–500, 1976.

Papper S: *Clinical Nephrology.* Boston, Little, Brown & Co, 1978.

Patwardhan RV, et al: Cimetidine spares the glucuronidation of lorazepam and oxazepam. *Gastroenterology* 79:912–916, 1980.

Petersen R, Ghoneim M: Diazepam and human memory: Influence on acquisition, retrieval, and state-dependent learning. *Prog Neuropsychophar-macol* 4:81–89, 1980.

Pevnick JS, Jasinski DR, Haertzen CA: Abrupt withdrawal from therapeuti-cally administered diazepam: Report of a case. *Arch Gen Psychiatry* 35:995–998, 1978.

Pitts FN, McClure JN: Lactate metabolism in anxiety neurosis. *N Engl J Med* 277:1329–1336, 1967.

Pleuvry BJ, Maddison SE, Odeh RB, et al: Respiratory and psychological ef-fects of oral temazepam in volunteers. *Br J Anaesth* 52:901–905, 1980.

Rao S, Sherbaniuk RW, Prasad K, et al: Cardiopulmonary effects of diaze-pam. *Clin Pharmacol Ther* 14:182–189, 1973.

Rosenbaum F: Anxiety, in Lazare A (ed): *Outpatient Psychiatry*. Baltimore, Williams & Wilkins Co, 1979, pp 252–256.

Roth T, Hartse KM, Saal PG et al: The effects of flurazepam lorazepam and triazolam on sleep and memory. *Psychopharmacology (Berlin)* 1980.

Salzman C: Antianxiety agents, in Crook T, Cohen G (eds): *Physicians' Hand-book on Psychotherapeutic Drug Use in the Aged*. New Canaan, Conn, Mark Powley Associates, Inc, 1981.

Scharf MB, Khosla N, Lysaght R, et al: Anterograde amnesia with oral loraze-pam. *J Clin Psychiatry* 44:362–364, 1983.

Schuckit MA: The diagnosis and treatment of panic and phobic states. *Fam Prac Recertification* 5:29–38, 1983.

Schuckit MA: Anxiety treatment: A commonsense approach. *Postgrad Med* 75:52–63, 1984.

Schumacher GE: Using pharmacokinetics in drug therapy. VII: Pharmacoki-netic factors influencing drug therapy in the aged. *Am J Pharmacol* 37:559–562, 1980.

Shader RI, Greenblatt DJ: Clinical implications of benzodiazepine pharmacoki-netics. *Am J Psychiatry* 134:652–655, 1977.

Steen SM, Amaha K, Martinez LR: Effect of oxazepam on respiratory response to carbon dioxide. *Curr Res Anaesth Analg* 45:455–458, 1966.

Utting HG, Pleuvry BJ: Benzoctamine — A study of the respiratory effects of oral doses in human volunteers and interactions with morphine in mice. *Br J Anaesth* 47:987–992, 1975.

Wallace S, et al: Factors affecting drug binding in plasma of elderly patients. *Br J Pharmacol* 3:327–330, 1976.

Wells CE: Pseudodementia. *Am J Psychiatry* 136:895–900, 1979.

Wilkinson GR, Schenker S: Drug disposition in liver disease. *Drug Metab Rev* 4:139–175, 1975.

Wilkinson GR, Schenker S: Effects of liver disease on drug disposition in man. *Biochem Pharmacol* 25:2675–2681, 1976.

CHAPTER 6

Alzheimer's Disease and Other Dementias

The prevalence of severe dementia in the United States has recently been estimated at about 1.3 million cases, of which 50% to 60% are of the Alzheimer's type (Terry and Katzman, 1983). An additional 2.8 million patients suffer mild to moderate impairment on the basis of cognitive decline. Over 10 billion of the 21 billion dollars spent on nursing home care in the United States in 1982 was expended on the care of patients with dementing illnesses. Roughly half of all nursing home beds are occupied by Alzheimer's victims and it is estimated that by the year 2030 the annual cost of taking care of Alzheimer's patients alone will exceed 30 billion dollars. Of those who are over age 65, 5% to 7% suffer from Alzheimer's disease; over age 80 it rises to 20%. As the number of our population living into old age continues to rise, the number of patients will correspondingly increase. In fact, Wells feels that we are about to face an epidemic of dementia (Wells, 1981).

DIAGNOSIS

The diagnosis of dementia can be made according to DSM-III criteria (Table 6-1). To make the diagnosis of dementia, one must observe a patient who has both memory impairment and a loss of other intellectual abilities of sufficient severity to interfere with social or occupational functioning. In addition, at least one of the following must be present: impairment of abstraction, impaired judgment, personality change, or other disturbances of higher cortical function such as aphasia, apraxia, agnosia, or constructional difficulty. In addition, the patient must not be delirious. If these criteria are met, we can make the diagnosis of dementia. This does not imply that we know the type

113

Table 6-1
Diagnostic Criteria for Alzheimer's Disease
(Primary Degenerative Dementia)

A. Dementia
  1. A loss of intellectual abilities of sufficient severity to interfere with social or occupational functioning

  2. Memory impairment

  3. At least one of the following:
    a. Impairment of abstract thinking (proverbs, similarities and differences, difficulty defining words and concepts)
    b. Impaired judgment
    c. Other disturbances of higher cortical function (aphasia, apraxia, agnosia, constructional difficulty)
    d. Personality change

  4. Clear consciousness, ie, not delirious

B. Insidious onset with uniformly progressive deteriorating course

C. Exclusion of all other specific causes of dementia by the history, physical examination, and laboratory tests

---

of dementing illness or what has caused the cognitive decline. It is analogous to making the diagnosis of pneumonia; we still need to find out the etiology or type of pneumonia.

To further make the diagnosis of Alzheimer's disease or primary degenerative dementia, the patient must have a dementing process, as defined above, with an insidious onset with a uniformly progressive deteriorating course. It is best to make the diagnosis of Alzheimer's disease based on the clinical course of the illness. Many clinicians are only familiar with the late stages of the disease and may fail to recognize earlier stages or attribute early changes to old age or senility. Reisberg et al (1982) have outlined superbly the clinical course of Alzheimer's disease (Table 6-2). Having a good idea of the natural history of the illness will not only aid in diagnosis but will also assist the caregivers in predicting what the future holds. In addition, it is likely that as treatments become available they will be more effective in the early stages of the illness and diagnostic considerations will become even more important.

Usually during the earliest stage of the illness, patients seem mildly forgetful and frequently complain of memory deficit; they may forget names or where they have placed household items. The patient may seem concerned, but has no social or employment problems and shows no evidence of memory deficit during a clinical interview. Benign senescent forgetfulness is a term commonly used to describe such complaints in elderly patients whose memory difficulties are not progressive.

The next stage of mild cognitive decline is evident by decreased performance in demanding employment or social situations. Patients complain of poor concentration, difficulty finding words and names, and may report that coworkers have noticed the patient's relatively poor performance. Some patients present initially with primarily visuospatial deficits and others may have difficulty with speech early in the course of the illness. Later, patients may get lost when traveling to an unfamiliar location. Anxiety and depression are common and many patients begin to deny symptoms.

Table 6-2
Stages of Alzheimer's Disease

Stage 1: No cognitive decline

Stage 2: Very mild cognitive decline
        Complaints of forgetfulness
        Forgets names
        Loses items
        No objective deficits in employment or social situations
        Patient displays appropriate concern

Stage 3: Mild cognitive decline
        May remember little of passage read from a book
        Decreased performance in demanding employment and social situations
        Coworkers become aware of patient's relatively poor performance
        Difficulty finding words and names
        May get lost when traveling to unfamiliar locations
        Anxiety is common
        Denial is likely

Stage 4: Moderate cognitive decline
        Clear-cut deficits
        Concentration deficits, eg, poor serial sevens
        Decreased knowledge of recent events in their lives and of current events
        Difficulties traveling alone and in handling personal finances
        Remains oriented to time and person
        Recognizes familiar persons and faces
        Can still travel to familiar locations, eg, corner drugstore
        Withdrawal from challenging situations
        Denial becomes dominant defense

Table 6-2 (continued)

Stage 5: Moderately severe cognitive decline
        Patient can no longer survive without some assistance
        May forget address or telephone number and names of close family members, eg, grandchildren
        Frequently disoriented to time or place
        Remembers own names and names of spouse and children
        May clothe themselves improperly, eg, shoe on wrong foot
        Need no assistance with eating or toileting

Stage 6: Severe cognitive decline
        Occasionally forgets spouse's name
        Largely unaware of all recent events and experiences in their lives
        Retain some sketchy knowledge of their past lives
        Unaware of surroundings, season, or year
        Sleep patterns frequently disturbed
        Personality and emotional changes frequent (often occur at earlier stages)
            Delusions, eg, spouse is an imposter, imaginary visitors, talks to own reflection in mirror
            Repetitive behaviors — continual cleaning, raking leaves, or lawn mowing
            Anxiety, agitation, occasional violent behavior
            Loss of initiative, abulia, apathy

Stage 7: Very severe cognitive decline
        Late dementia
        Inability to communicate, grunting
        Incontinent of urine
        Needs assistance with toileting and eating
        May be unable to walk
        Focal neurologic signs and symptoms common

As the illness progresses, patients become unable to travel alone and are unable to handle their personal finances. Memory for recent events will be drastically impaired, and patients display decreased knowledge of current events. Complex tasks are impossible, but patients remain well oriented to time and person and can travel to very familiar places like the corner drugstore. Many patients are aware of their deficits and are capable of understanding what is happening to them. Patients instinctively withdraw from previously challenging situations. Denial may be pronounced.

During the next phase, patients can no longer survive without some assistance, are unable to recall major relevant aspects of their current lives, and may be unable to recall names of close friends or even family members. Delusions are common. The spouse may be accused of being an imposter or the patient may talk to imaginary persons or to his own reflection in the mirror. Depression, agitation, and violent behavior may occur. Frequently patients are disoriented to time or place. They generally require no assistance with toileting or eating, but may have difficulty choosing the proper clothing to wear; they may put their shoes on the wrong feet, for instance.

The last stages of the disease finds patients totally incapacitated and disoriented. They eventually forget their own names and may not recognize their spouse. Incontinence is common. Personality and emotional changes become very pronounced in this stage but occasionally occur even in the earliest stages. Eventually all verbal abilities are lost, motor skills deteriorate, and patients require total care. At this stage, generalized cortical and focal neurologic signs and symptoms are frequently present. Death usually occurs from total debilitation or infection.

The course of Alzheimer's disease varies from two to as long as 20 years from onset to death. The average is six to eight years. Typically, the illness progresses at a fairly constant rate. That is, if it has progressed rapidly over the past year it is likely to continue at that rate. A slowly progressive illness over the past five to 10 years means that the patient may survive for a number of years. These are not infallible rules, but do serve as a rough guideline (Jenike, 1985a).

TREATABLE CAUSES OF DEMENTIA

Dementia can be caused by a variety of disorders. Haase (1977) listed over 50 diseases that may cause dementia, and this list is constantly growing. Alzheimer's disease is, however, the overwhelmingly dominant disorder producing dementia in the elderly, with postmortem studies confirming that between 50% and 60% of all cases of dementia have classic Alzheimer's changes (Jellinger, 1976; Sourander and Sjogren, 1970; Tomlinson et al, 1968; 1970). Other neurologic diseases produce the picture of dementia: Parkinson's disease (about a third become demented), Huntington's chorea, and Creutzfeldt-Jakob. After Alzheimer's disease, however, multiple strokes, or so-called multi-infarct dementia is the second leading cause of dementing illness. Hachinski and colleagues have developed a group of questions that can assist the clinician and researcher in ruling out multi-infarct dementia (Hachinski et al, 1974) (Table 6-3).

Once the diagnosis of dementia has been made, the clinician must perform a thorough medical, neurologic, and psychiatric evaluation. *Brain failure requires as thorough an evaluation as heart failure or renal*

Table 6-3
Hachinski Ischemic Score

Feature	Score	Present	Absent
1. Abrupt onset	2	____	____
2. Stepwise deterioration	1	____	____
3. Fluctuating course	2	____	____
4. Nocturnal confusion	1	____	____
5. Relative preservation of personality	1	____	____
6. Depression	1	____	____
7. Somatic complaints	1	____	____
8. Emotional incontinence	1	____	____
9. History of hypertension	1	____	____
10. History of strokes	2	____	____
11. Evidence of associated atherosclerosis	1	____	____
12. Focal neurologic symptoms	2	____	____
13. Focal neurologic signs	2	____	____
Total Score	____		

A total score of 5 or greater is suggestive of multi-infarct dementia.

Adapted from Hachinski et al: Cerebral blood flow in dementia. *Arch Neurol* 32:632-637, 1975.

failure. Some potentially treatable causes of dementia are listed in Table 6-4. A suggested workup of a demented patient to eliminate most treatable etiologies is listed in Table 6-5 (Jenike, 1982a). One of the most common causes of a treatable dementia is the use of drugs. Almost any drug can cause cognitive impairment. Propranolol has been reported to mimic Alzheimer's disease. Other common offenders include methyldopa, clonidine, haloperidol, chlorpromazine, phenytoin, bromides, paraldehyde, primidone, phenacetin, phenobarbital, cimetidine, quinidine, procainamide, disopyramide, and atropine and related compounds. A trial without medication is the only way to determine if a drug is a factor. Often alcoholic patients will show greatly improved cognition when they stop drinking.

Tumors may cause cognitive impairment either directly by interfering with the CNS or by a poorly understood remote effect. Such remote effects are associated with pulmonary neoplasms in the great majority of cases, but other reported sites include the ovary, breast, rectum, and prostate.

Thyroid abnormalities, both hyper- and hypothyroid states, are the most common endocrine dysfunctions associated with cognitive impairment. Unless replacement therapy is started early, irreversible deficits may occur.

Vitamin B_{12} deficiency may present as dementia, depression, or

Table 6-4
Potentially Treatable Causes of Dementia

1. Drugs and alcohol	Beta-blockers, methyldopa, clonidine, haloperidol, chlorpromazine, phenytoin, bromides, phenobarbitol, cimetidine, steroids, procainamide, disopyramide phosphate, atropine, alcohol (a trial without drugs or alcohol is needed)
2. Tumors	Direct CNS invasion; remote effect, mostly lung, occasionally ovary, prostate, rectum, breast
3. Nutritional	Vitamin B_{12} deficiency (dementia may precede anemia), folate deficiency, pellagra, Wernicke-Korsakoff encephalopathy
4. Infection	Syphilis, abscess, encephalitis
5. Metabolic	Electrolyte disturbances; hepatic, renal disease; chronic obstructive lung disease
6. Inflammatory	Lupus erythematosus
7. Endocrine	Thyroid abnormalities (hypo- and hyperthyroid states); adrenal, parathyroid abnormalities
8. Trauma	Subdural hematoma
9. Psychiatric/ neurologic	Schizophrenia, seizures, normal pressure hydrocephalus (dementia, ataxia, incontinence), depression (most common, may need treatment trial)

anergia. These disturbances may precede the anemia. Approximately three quarters of pernicious anemia patients have objective memory impairment and 60% have abnormal EEGs. Most return to normal after replacement therapy. All "senile" patients should be screened for megaloblastic anemia, and serum B_{12} levels should be checked on all patients with unexplained dementia, especially when they have persistent fatigue or a history of gastric surgery. Folic acid deficiency may also present as megaloblastic anemia with dementia. Prior to starting folic acid replacement, the serum B_{12} level should be checked. These levels tend to fall when folic acid therapy is started, and this could precipitate or aggravate neurological disturbances in patients with undiagnosed pernicious anemia (Lishman, 1978).

Neurosyphilis, which may progress to frank dementia, if untreated, is frequently associated with concentration difficulty, faulty judgment, emotional instability, and malaise. In older persons the VDRL and FTA-ABS tests are both done as serologic studies for syphilis. The FTA-

Table 6-5
Workup of the Dementing Patient

1. History from patient *and* relative or friend
2. Mental status examination
3. Physical examination with vital signs
4. Neurologic examination
5. CT scan and EEG
6. Thyroid function tests; serum B_{12} and folic acid determinations
7. Chest x-ray, ECG
8. Complete blood count, urinanalysis, glucose, BUN, Ca, serum albumin, electrolytes, alkaline phosphatase, VDRL and FTA, sedimentation rate.

Others (as indicated)
1. Drug levels
2. Toxic screen
3. Brain scan
4. Lumbar puncture (*not routinely*)

ABS is more specific and important because of the frequency of serum negative VDRL tests for tertiary syphilis in older people. A negative VDRL but positive FTA-ABS calls for cerebrospinal fluid serologies to establish or rule out tertiary syphilis (O'Daniel et al, 1981).

Subdural hematomas usually follow head trauma, but may occur spontaneously in the elderly, especially in patients with blood dyscrasias or those on anticoagulants. Patients with a chronic subdural hematoma may present with increasing difficulty with concentration, memory lapses, and fluctuating level of consciousness. Variability in the mental state from day to day and even from hour to hour is often the most important indicator of this condition. Sometimes headache or episodes of restlessness may occur. The EEG is abnormal in 90% of these patients. A CT scan may show a mass effect, but the subdural hematoma assumes the same density as brain tissue approximately ten days after a bleed. After that, a brain scan is the most useful diagnostic test (Lishman, 1978).

The erythrocyte sedimentation rate (ESR) is a quick, inexpensive screening test for inflammatory conditions, especially collagen vascular diseases which may present with the picture of dementia.

Normal pressure hydrocephalus is characterized by the development over many weeks or months of memory impairment, physical and mental slowness, unsteadiness of gait, and urinary incontinence. The mental changes usually occur first, although gait disturbance may be the presenting symptom. Urinary incontinence generally appears much later. These patients should be referred for a complete neurologic work-up including a CT scan and *Risa* cisternography which may show characteristically dilated ventricles with abnormalities of cerebrospinal flow (Wells, 1977).

Another very important reversible dementia is the pseudodementia of depression. As many as 7% of demented patients are found to be depressed, with the dementia resolving after proper treatment of the depression (Wells, 1977). While it is difficult to differentiate pseudodementia from true dementia without a trial of electroconvulsive therapy or medication, some clinical points may be helpful. First, the onset of endogenous depression is typically acute and recent, whereas that of dementia is usually insidious. Second, in depression there is no decline in abilities or memory until the appearance of depressive symptoms. Third, the depressed patient will frequently communicate a sense of distress, whereas in primary dementia the emotions tend to be shallow. Finally, the demented patient may tend to confabulate while the depressed patient is more likely to counter most questions by "I don't know!" (Wells, 1979).

There is some controversy about the use of CT scans in the workup of the demented patient. Such a scan costs less than a one-day stay in the hospital, and can be a very important part of the workup of the demented patient. The CT scan may help diagnose the cause of reversible and/or treatable dementias, such as subdural hematoma, normal pressure hydrocephalus, and brain tumor. It may also make apparent less treatable etiologies such as multiple strokes or Alzheimer's disease. In the latter the CT scan would show *marked* cortical atrophy with widened sulci and shrunken gyri, and ventricular dilatation. Mild to moderate cortical atrophy is not well correlated with brain pathology or clinical condition (Lishman, 1978; Wells, 1977).

THE DEXAMETHASONE SUPPRESSION TEST AND DEMENTIA

One of the common clinical dilemmas facing the physician who treats elderly patients is the separation of the truly demented patient from the patient who has reversible cognitive impairment on the basis of depression, ie, pseudodementia. If the dexamethasone suppression test (DST) could be shown to be normal in mild dementia and frequently abnormal in depression, the test could be used as a diagnostic aid.

Numerous studies indicate that the DST may be useful in identifying patients with depressive illness (Carroll et al, 1981; Schlesser et al, 1980; Jenike, 1981; 1982b; 1982c; 1983a) and in following their response to treatment (Jenike, 1983a). While advanced age alone apparently does not alter the utility of the overnight DST (Tourigny-Rivard et al, 1981), its efficacy in elderly patients with Alzheimer's disease has been questioned. In particular, it has been reported that patients with dementia of the Alzheimer's type who are not depressed frequently have abnormal DST results. Spar and Gerner found that nine of 17 Alzheimer's patients had abnormal DST results (Spar and Gerner, 1982), while Raskind et al (1982) reported that seven of 15 patients had abnormal values. However, an examination of the data suggests that both groups of patients were moderately to severely demented. Spar and Gerner's patients had a mean Mini-Mental State Exam score of 13.3 (out of a possible score of 30) and had been ill for an average of 4.3 years. The patients of Raskind et al had no correct responses to the Short Portable Mental Status Questionnaire and a mean duration of illness of 7.4 years. Thus, it may be that the abnormal DST results are caused by *advanced* disease. Most patients for whom the diagnostic confusion between depression and dementia is a problem are only mildly demented. Several case reports suggest that the DST may be helpful in this differential diagnosis. Rudorfer and Clayton reported a patient with pseudodementia whose abnormal DST result normalized after treatment of the underlying depressive illness (Rudorfer and Clayton, 1981). Greden and Carroll (1979) described a catatonic patient with an initial diagnosis of dementia who had an abnormal DST result. As a result of this finding, a diagnosis of primary unipolar depression was entertained, and electroconvulsive therapy (ECT) was begun. Her initially abnormal DST result returned to normal following two courses of ECT. Similarly, McAllister et al (1982) reported two patients for whom the DST appeared to be useful in distinguishing depression accompanied by cognitive dysfunction from dementia.

A recent report of 18 well-characterized Alzheimer's patients, who were separated into two groups on the basis of their degree of impairment, found that of 13 patients with mild cognitive impairment, only one had a slightly abnormal DST result (Jenike and Albert, 1984). In contrast, four of the five more advanced patients had grossly abnormal DSTs. These differences were found to be highly significant. None of the patients were depressed according to clinical interview and Hamilton Depression Rating Scale. These data indicate that the DST may be useful for identifying persons with treatable depression among those with mild cognitive dysfunction. The results further suggest that as Alzheimer's disease progresses, the DST no longer can be used as a neuroendocrine correlate of depression. The most likely explanation for the increasing incidence of abnormal DST results among moderately to severely impaired patients is the impact on hypothalamic function of the neurochemical and neuropathologic changes associated with Alzheimer's disease (Davies, 1979). However, it remains possible that the depression in Alzheimer's patients presents in an unusual fashion. Thus, patients with abnormal DST results and low Hamilton Depression Rating Scale scores may, in fact, be depressed. Only if such patients are treated for depression can this possibility be ruled out.

It is hoped that future work will clarify these issues, since depressive pseudodementia is one of the most common causes of reversible cognitive change in the elderly.

THEORIES OF ETIOLOGY

Four main theories of the cause of Alzheimer's disease predominate: genetic, viral, aluminum, and immune. The etiologic factor (or factors) is not known. Some of the relevant findings in reference to each theory will be reviewed.

Genetic

Relatives of patients diagnosed as having Alzheimer's disease commonly ask if the disorder is inherited. The answer to this question remains elusive. Rarely, a family is identified where the illness appears as if it were a straightforward dominant condition (Terry and Katzman, 1983; Cook et al, 1979; Goudsmit et al, 1981). There is growing evidence that the younger the age of onset of the disease, the more likely a sibling is to develop the disease. With late onset illness, the risk to first-degree relatives is increased little, if at all (Heston et al, 1981; Mortimer and Schuman, 1981; Larsson et al, 1963). Twin studies have yielded conflicting results. Incomplete concordance among identical twins is reported (Jarvik et al, 1971; 1980). However, another report of identical twins who developed Alzheimer's disease over 12 years apart casts doubt on the supposed lack of concordance in twins (Cook et al, 1981). Perhaps if one twin develops the illness, the other will also if followed long enough. This case implies that factors other than genetics may influence the age of onset of the disease.

Further evidence for a genetic involvement comes from the finding that apparently all patients with Down's syndrome, a genetic disorder, develop changes consistent with Alzheimer's disease if they reach age 35 to 40. They invariably show significant numbers of plaques and tangles in cerebral cortex and hippocampus (Owens et al, 1971; Burger and Vogel, 1973; Heston, 1976).

These findings make the genetic theory particularly attractive, especially for the occasional familial cases.

Viral

It is now well documented that other degenerative neurologic illnesses, such as kuru (Gajdusek and Zigos, 1957) and Creutzfeld-Jacob disease (Roos et al, 1973) in man and scrapie (Hourrigan et al, 1979) and transmissable mink encephalopathy (Marsh et al, 1974) in animals, are caused by viruses or other subcellular infective agents like prions (Prusiner, 1984). It has also been demonstrated that certain strains of the scrapie agent inoculated into the CNS of certain recipient mouse strains induce the formation of neuritic plaques very much like those of Alzheimer's disease, except for an absence of paired helical filaments (Bruce and Fraser, 1975).

A number of trials have been made in an effort to transmit an infective agent from man to primates. These have all met with no success (Terry and Katzman, 1983; Gibbs and Gajdusek, 1978), with the exception of one report where specimens from two of six patients with familial Alzheimer's disease induced a spongy encephalopathy in recipient primates (Gibbs and Gajdusek, 1978). This report has, however, been retracted (Terry and Katzman, 1983).

In another report, an extract of brain tissue from patients with Alzheimer's disease seemed to induce the formation of paired helical filaments in cultured human fetal neurons (DeBoni and Crapper, 1978). These researchers reportedly now feel that this was a degenerative toxic phenomenon in the recipient cultures rather than a change related to the inoculum (Terry and Katzman, 1983).

Viral theories remain of interest, but there is still no hard evidence that viruses are involved in the transmission of Alzheimer's disease.

Aluminum

Aluminum intoxication as a possible etiologic agent gained attention when it was discovered that rabbits exposed to toxic amounts of aluminum developed neurofibrillary tangles (Klatzo et al, 1965; Cummings and Benson, 1983). These tangles were, however, somewhat different from those found in the brains of Alzheimer's patients (Terry and Pena, 1965). Some investigators (Crapper et al, 1973: 1976) found elevated brain aluminum levels in Alzheimer's patients, while other studies have failed to confirm an elevation (McDermott et al, 1977; 1979). Others (Delaney, 1979; Shore et al, 1980) found normal cerebrospinal fluid (CSF) and serum aluminum levels, while Markesbery and colleagues reported that intraneuronal aluminum content was also normal (Markesbery et al, 1981).

Dialysis dementia is a disease known to be associated with significantly elevated levels of brain aluminum; neurofibrillary tangles, however, are not found (Dunea et al, 1978; Lederman and Henry, 1978; Rozas et al, 1978). Others find no differences in brain aluminum content between Alzheimer's patients and age-matched controls. They do, however, find increased brain aluminum content associated with aging (McDermott et al, 1977; 1979). The neurofibrillary tangles induced experimentally by aluminum administration differ from those of Alzheimer's disease in that they are straight rather than twisted and they are distributed in the brainstem and spinal cord instead of the cortex (Yates, 1979).

Thus it appears that the weight of the cumulative evidence is against the likelihood that aluminum is the agent responsible for Alzheimer's disease (Cummings and Benson, 1983).

Immune Function

Immune function abnormalities have been reported in Alzheimer's patients. One group (Behan and Feldman, 1970) reported that two thirds of their patients had serum protein abnormalities which included decreases in albumin and increases in α-2-macroglobulin, α-1-antitrypsin, and haptoglobin fractions. Others (Jonker et al, 1982) report normal CSF immunoglobulin levels. Impaired cellular immune responses (Behan and Behan, 1979) as well as impaired immunoregulation (Miller et al, 1981) have been observed. Elevated levels of brain antibody have also been reported in Alzheimer's patients (Nandy, 1978).

Neuritic (senile) plaques have an amyloid core which some investigators think is composed of antigen-antibody complexes catabolized by phagocytes and degraded by lysosomes (Wisniewski et al, 1970; Wisniewski and Terry, 1973; Roth et al, 1966). Altered immune function could explain the presence of amyloid in senile plaques and its occasional occurrence in cerebral vessels (Glenner, 1978). At present, it is unknown whether these immunologic abnormalities are primary and thus of etiologic significance, or secondary to some more basic process (Cummings and Benson, 1983).

Thus far, no peculiarities of histocompatibility antigens have been found among Alzheimer's patients (Henschke et al, 1978; Sulkava et al, 1980; Whalley et al, 1980). Although the immune hypothesis is conceptually of interest, there is insufficient evidence to draw any definite conclusions at present.

PRINCIPLES OF MANAGEMENT

Once treatable causes for dementia have been ruled out, the primary care physician must manage a patient with a chronic and progressive illness. The physician will be required to be familiar with the use of psychoactive drugs in the elderly and will be asked to counsel and advise family members. Many physicians prefer not to manage such patients and referral to another colleague or geriatric specialist is encouraged under these circumstances (Jenike, 1985a).

Management must involve family members who may choose to keep the dementing patient at home until very late in the course of the illness and it is not uncommon for a spouse to devote almost the entire day to caring for the patient. A number of drugs are now available as potential memory enhancers. Although none are dramatically effective, family members will ask about them. Drugs are available to treat depression, psychosis, and behavioral problems in dementing individuals. There are also a number of agencies which can be of major assistance to physicians, patients, and families of Alzheimer's victims. These issues will be reviewed individually.

Drugs for Memory Enhancement

A wide variety of pharmacologic agents have been investigated for the treatment of cognitive decline in Alzheimer's disease.

Less than a decade ago we assumed that arteriosclerotic narrowing was the primary pathology responsible for Alzheimer's and a number of cerebral vasodilators and anticoagulants were tried in an effort to dilate stenotic vessels. With the finding that most patients had fairly normal vessels, these approaches were discontinued.

In the past few years, new discoveries have stimulated innovative pharmacologic approaches based on the cholinergic hypothesis of memory. This hypothesis is based on a number of findings: (1) anticholinergic drugs, such as scopolamine, induce memory deficits in healthy young subjects similar to those observed in nondemented elderly subjects; (2) these deficits are reversed by physostigmine, a cholinergic agent that potentiates synaptic acetylcholine; (3) cholinergic drugs such as arecholine and physostigmine improve aspects of learning and memory in normal subjects; (4) cholinergic neurons are found to be selectively destroyed in autopsy studies of Alzheimer's brains; and (5) the activity of choline acetyltransferase, the enzyme which catalyzes the synthesis of acetylcholine, is reduced in brain tissue obtained from patients with Alzheimer's disease (Bartus et al, 1982). Because of these cholinergic deficits, many cholinergic enhancers have been used in an attempt to bolster this failing system. Patients and their families frequently ask about choline and lecithin and some take lecithin which they have purchased from so-called health-food stores. Unfortunately, these cholinergic precursors have not been useful; there is no clinical change in most patients. Studies with other drugs, however, that stimulate cholinergic transmission are more encouraging. Physostigmine, now available for research purposes in an oral form, does improve cognitive test scores in some patients, but its overall clinical effect is less dramatic, and its effect on the progression of Alzheimer's disease remains to be determined (Thal et al, 1983).

A group of drugs have been classified loosely as metabolic enhancers. Hydergine remains the most commonly prescribed drug for Alzheimer's patients and a number of controlled studies have shown minimal improvement with Hydergine. Hydergine consists of three hydrogenated alkaloids of ergot, has a 30-year history of use, and has been shown to be extremely safe, even with long-term administration (Spiegel et al, 1983).

There are at least 12 placebo-controlled studies which have compared Hydergine either with placebo alone or with placebo and papaverine (Bazo, 1973; Rosen, 1975; Rehman, 1973; McConnachie, 1973. Thibault, 1974; Banen, 1972; Rao and Norris, 1972; Jennings, 1972; Triboletti and Ferri, 1969; Ditch et al, 1971; Gerin, 1969; Roubicek et al, 1972). Thirteen of 36 behavioral variables assessed showed a statistically significant improvement with Hydergine in at least 50% of the studies. The variables that improved significantly were mental alertness, orientation, confusion, recent memory, depression, emotional lability, anxiety, fear, motivation, initiative, agitation, vertigo, and locomotion; overall impression and global therapeutic change also showed significant improvement. The variable that showed the most significant change was depression. Thus, two recent reviews have concluded that most studies with Hydergine show a small but measurable improvement on some variables (Reisberg et al, 1981; Hollister and Yesavage, 1984). Hollister and Yesavage also noted that in their clinical experience an occasional patient shows a dramatic response to the drug.

A review of the literature suggests guidelines for duration of treatment and dose level of Hydergine. Studies that used a treatment trial of several months were clearly more likely to show improvement than treatment trials of a shorter duration, and recent evidence indicates that a six-month course of drug may be most beneficial (Hollister and Yesavage, 1984). While doses of 3.0 to 4.5 mg/day have most often been employed in American studies of Hydergine, 6 mg/day is commonly used in Europe, and doses as large as 12 mg/day have been given without serious side effects (Hollister and Yesavage, 1984). This suggests that it may be reasonable to use doses considerably larger than those previously used. In summary, individual effects are generally small and the variable that showed the most significant change was depression (Rosen, 1975; Thibault, 1974; Banen, 1972; Jennings, 1972; Ditch et al, 1971; Reisberg et al, 1981). Even though study results are weak, experienced clinicians occasionally report an individual patient with a good response to a three- to six-month trial of this agent. If there is no improvement after six months, Hydergine should be discontinued.

Piracetam, another metabolic enhancer, may influence cerebral energy reserves and increase the ratio of adenosine triphosphate (ATP) to adenosine diphosphate (ADP) in the brain. There is preliminary evidence that piracetam and related drugs may be useful in improving functioning in patients with mild to moderate senile dementia, but not in severely demented patients. More research is needed to see if clinically significant results are obtained (Reisberg et al, 1981; Crook and Cohen, 1981).

Psychostimulants, such as methylphenidate hydrochloride, may improve mood in depressed demented patients, but do not enhance cognition. Procaine hydrochloride, which inhibits MAO activity has similar actions. There is some research in progress looking at the effectiveness of vasopressin and its analogs on memory in Alzheimer's patients. Vasopressin and other brain peptides, such as ACTH and melanocyte-stimulating hormone (MSH), have been shown to affect the learning process, particularly in animals (Reisberg et al, 1981).

Even though the body of basic information about Alzheimer's has increased dramatically in the last few years, the pharmacologic treatment remains in its infancy. Research has thus far produced no consistently effective agents which the primary care physician can use to treat Alzheimer's patients. It is likely, however, that breakthroughs will occur in the next decade. All patients with mild or moderate Alzheimer's should be referred to research centers for experimental protocols when this is feasible.

Chelation Therapy

Chelation therapy is offered by an estimated 1000 practitioners and clinics in the United States and these clinics frequently announce that they can treat angina, reverse atherosclerosis, reverse blindness, open blocked arteries, dissolve kidney stones, dissolve small cataracts, reduce arthritis symptoms, decrease the effects of aging, and improve memory. Many families of Alzheimer's victims inquire into these treatments and understandably will invest huge sums of money in the hope that some benefit will be forthcoming (*The Harvard Medical School Health Letter*, July 1984).

Before chelation therapy is begun, most centers proceed with an expensive battery of tests which may exceed $1000 in cost. These rarely serve to disqualify a willing candidate. The treatment consists of 30 to 40 sessions in which the chemical EDTA is given intravenously over three or four hours. These sessions are generally spread out over eight to 10 weeks with intervening periods of "rest." Since EDTA binds to a variety of dissolved minerals or metals present in the body to form a complex which is renally excreted, it is very useful if one is suffering from heavy-metal poisoning, such as lead poisoning.

Advocates of chelation therapy have come up with a number of vague and highly improbable theories which have never been subjected to rigorous testing (Jenike, 1984b). All of the evidence in favor of chelation therapy is in the form of anecdotes or uncontrolled trials. A course of chelation therapy costs from $3000 to $6000 and is not covered by insurance providers.

After reviewing the available information on chelation therapy for heart disease and other ailments, the editors of a distinguished newsletter (*The Harvard Medical School Health Letter*, July 1984) reached the following conclusions: (1) there is no credible evidence that chelation therapy works as claimed; (2) there is good theoretical reason to think that it does not work, except as an elaborate placebo; and (3) as a placebo, the treatment is very expensive and, far from being unprofitable, chelation can afford quite a high income to those who promote it.

We have seen a number of patients who have been urged to undergo chelation therapy for Alzheimer's disease. Proponents of the therapy feel that chelation somehow acts as a vasodilator and increases blood flow to the brain. This rationale seems particularly illogical in light of the fact that most Alzheimer's patients have normal cerebral vessels and that the pathology of Alzheimer's disease is no longer thought to be secondary to brain vascular insufficiency.

Until controlled scientific studies have demonstrated some benefit, it seems unreasonable to recommend chelation therapy, particularly in light of the significant cost and doubtful benefit to the individual patient.

Drugs to Control Psychiatric Symptoms

Some Alzheimer's victims will suffer from concomitant behavioral abnormalities, depression, psychosis, and/or anxiety. Most Alzheimer's patients do not suffer from the illness of depression and it is not inevitable in the course of the disease. When present, depression and anxiety can be treated effectively in the demented patient. In each patient, depression should be sought and when identified should be treated vigorously (see chapter 4). Secondary amines with relatively low anticholinergic activity such as desipramine and nortriptyline or newer agents such as trazodone and maprotiline should be the drugs of first choice. In a patient who is not sleeping well trazodone or nortriptyline, given at bedtime, may assist with sleep. In patients who are hypersomnic, daytime doses of desipramine may help activate the patient (Jenike, 1983b; 1985b).

Some patients who do not respond to standard antidepressants may respond to monoamine oxidase inhibitors (MAOIs) (Jenike, 1984a; 1985b; 1985c). It has recently been demonstrated that there is a marked increase in MAO levels with age in human plasma, platelets, and brain (Robinson et al, 1972; Robinson, 1975; Horita, 1978). The recent finding that demented patients have even higher MAO levels than age-matched controls makes the use of MAO inhibitors to treat depression in Alzheimer's victims even more inviting (Gottfries et al, 1983; Jenike, 1985c). The following two cases illustrate the beneficial results of aggressive pharmacologic treatment of patients with concomitant major depression and Alzheimer's disease. Both patients failed to respond to standard agents but improved greatly when an MAO inhibitor was begun.

Case 1: Mrs. A is a 73-year-old woman who has had progressive memory deficit, typical of Alzheimer's disease, for the past four years. A workup to rule out treatable causes for her cognitive decline was completely normal with the exception of her CT scan which showed moderate cortical atrophy. Her Dementia Rating Scale (Mattis, 1976) score was 125 out of a possible 144 which placed her in the category of mild dementia (Jenike and Albert, 1984). Other neuropsychologic tests were completely consistent with the diagnosis of Alzheimer's disease. Mrs. A herself had no history of depression, but her father had suffered numerous depressive episodes. Her family psychiatric history was otherwise negative.

At interview, Mrs. A admitted to dysphoric feelings and appeared on the verge of tears. She had lost interest in work, hobbies, and social activities and felt lethargic throughout the day. Her appetite had decreased and she had recently lost about 10 lbs. She had to force herself to eat. She had no psychotic symptoms, but intermittently felt hopeless and had become very obsessive.

She had been depressed for over a year and numerous medication trials had failed. On amitriptyline and nortriptyline she failed to improve with low doses and developed an anticholinergic delirium at higher doses. Maprotiline, desipramine, and methylphenidate were of no help and alprazolam worsened her symptoms. The patient did not remember the medication dosages and her old records could not be located. They were, however, administered by an experienced geriatric psychiatrist.

She was begun on tranylcypromine 10 mg twice a day. Her daughter called the next week to report a dramatic improvement in her mother's mood and activity level. Over the next two weeks her appetite improved and she gained 5 lbs. Two weeks later she was beginning to feel slightly more depressed and tranylcypromine was gradually increased to 20 mg twice daily with rapid improvement. Her daughter states that the change in her mother's mood has allowed her to lead a much happier and independent life despite her progressive memory loss. Six months later, Mrs. A continues to be active and socially involved.

Case 2: Mr. B, a 68-year-old retired laborer, was evaluated for a one-year history of worsening memory. He had also become increasingly withdrawn and was losing interest in his past hobbies— traveling and reading. His daughter frequently found him sitting alone in the dark. He had stopped driving, had lost his appetite with a resultant 14-lb weight loss, and seemed frequently confused with inability to concentrate. He felt very hopeless and depressed. His mother had, on one occasion, received ECT for severe depression with good result and his older brother had been chronically depressed with at least one episode of psychotic depression requiring hospitalization. Mr. B denied a history of depressive episodes and his daughter confirmed that he had always been a very active and optimistic person.

Mr. B's neuropsychological tests were consistent with Alzheimer's disease. His Dementia Rating Scale score was 135 out of a possible 144 and all other neuropsychological tests were consistent with the diagnosis of Alzheimer's disease. It was clear that he also suffered from a superimposed disabling depression. Treatable causes for cognitive decline were ruled out.

Mr. B was begun on desipramine, 25 mg at bedtime, and the dose was increased slowly to 200 mg daily. He suffered no side effects, but also got no better over the next six weeks despite measured blood levels in the therapeutic range. Desipramine eventually was discontinued and nortriptyline was begun, again starting with low dosage. Once again he failed to respond despite a blood level measurement in the therapeutic range.

Since Mr. B had not improved on two antidepressants, and the family feared ECT, a MAOI was begun. After a ten-day drug-free period, tranylcypromine was started at 10 mg twice a day and slowly increased to 20 mg twice daily. After two weeks, Mr. B was much improved and within six weeks described himself as being "back to my former self" despite his persistent cognitive deficits. At eight-month follow-up, he remains affectively stable despite considerable cognitive decline.

Standard tricyclic antidepressants were not effective in either patient. These agents, even when effective, have several drawbacks when used in depressed and demented elderly patients. Anticholinergic effects, both peripherally (tachycardia, constipation, urinary retention, and dry mouth) and centrally (confusion and delirium), are particularly troublesome in elderly patients. In addition, as previously mentioned, it is now well documented that central cholinergic deficits exist in Alzheimer's patients which may make these patients particularly prone to developing further memory impairment and cognitive decline when such drugs are used (Goodnick and Gershon, 1984). MAO inhibitors, on the other hand, do not produce clinically significant central or peripheral anticholinergic effects. If the main side effects, orthostatic hypotension and insomnia, are tolerable, these drugs can be used safely in elderly patients when certain dietary precautions are observed (see chapter 4). Neither of our two patients developed orthostatic changes.

Sometimes moderate doses of methylphenidate (10 to 40 mg/d) may help motivate and energize a demented patient (see chapter 4). If there is no response within a few days, it should be discontinued. Similarly, behavioral disturbances and psychosis can usually be managed effectively in this population. Low doses (ie, 0.5 mg twice daily initially) of a high potency neuroleptic, such as haloperidol or fluphenazine, may allow many patients to live at home who would otherwise have to be managed in chronic care facilities or in state psychiatric institutions (see chapter 3). Patients with preexisting movement disorders, such as Parkinson's disease, may be better treated with very low doses of thioridazine (ie, 10 mg twice daily initially). Low potency neuroleptics like thioridazine are more likely to cause excessive sedation, anticholinergic effects (tachycardia, urinary retention, dry mouth, confusion, etc), and orthostatic hypotension, but are less likely to cause parkinsonian side effects than the high potency drugs (see chapter 3).

Management of the Family

Family members may well react to the fact that their relative has Alzheimer's disease as the worst news they have ever received. Family members who have a pre-existing psychiatric illness may decompensate and the primary care physician may have to contact the treating psychotherapist to coordinate care. Many family members will have suspected the diagnosis and may be relieved to have an understanding physician who will be available and helpful over the course of the illness. Family members may be stunned initially and ask few questions. Information should not be forced upon them. Careful explanation about any further evaluative tests should be given and a follow-up appointment within a week should be arranged. Common questions include:

How long will my husband live? Will she deteriorate rapidly? A child may ask what his chances are of developing the disease — is it hereditary? Is there a treatment?

Within the first few weeks of making the diagnosis, family members should see a social worker who is aware of community resources such as visiting nurse availability, meals-on-wheels, financial resources, and nursing home procedures. For the very early Alzheimer's patient, this may seem premature, but family members will be reassured by the knowledge that help will be available when needed in the future. Most families read about the illness and become acutely aware of the devastating course of the illness.

Legal consultation is mandatory as financial ruin may result if finances are not handled appropriately. Some states allow transfer of funds from an afflicted individual to other family members, but long waiting periods may be required to get government financial assistance.

Even with a compassionate and empathetic physician, many families feel alone with this illness and are unable to find friends who understand. Embarrassment may make them withdraw from previous social contacts. To meet the need for communication and information, families in many areas have established volunteer organizations which are involved in helping each other, sharing solutions to management problems, exchanging information, supporting needed legislation and research, and educating the community. These organizations welcome members who are concerned about all of the dementing illnesses, of which Alzheimer's disease is the most common. The number of such support groups is growing rapidly and families consistently rave about how helpful they are. These groups offer friendship, information about the diseases, information about resources and local doctors, and they give members the opportunity to exchange ideas.

These local volunteer organizations have established a national organization, the Alzheimer's Disease and Related Disorders Association (ADRDA), whose goals are family support, education, advocacy, and encouraging research. The address of ADRDA is: 360 N. Michigan Avenue, Chicago, IL 60601. The national organization will give family members the addresses of local groups.

Each family member should be encouraged to read one of the available lay books on Alzheimer's disease. *The 36-Hour Day* is required reading for anyone (including physicians) who is dealing with an individual with a progressive dementing illness (Mace and Rabins, 1981).

Families need to be encouraged to maintain a structured, predictable environment for the patient. Any change can be devastating and stressful to a demented patient and may produce a so-called catastrophic reaction, ie, a massive emotional overresponse to minor stress. A schedule in which activities such as arising, eating, medication-taking, and exercise occur at the same time each day maximizes the patient's familiarity with his personal environment. At times an orientation center with pertinent information such as the date, time, schedule of household events, and pictures of relevant people is very helpful.

Guilt, unrealistic expectations, and assumption of excessive responsibility are common responses of families (Rabins et al, 1982; Rabins, 1984). In discussing these and similar issues, the physician should focus both on physical realities and on the family's emotional responses to the patient. One frequently encountered source of difficulty is that the care of an elderly person often represents a reversal of parent/child roles. There is no one way to handle such problems and physicians may try to avoid such discussions for fear that they may not know how to handle the conflicts. In the overwhelming majority of such cases, however, just allowing family members to discuss these and other issues will be therapeutic in and of itself.

Certain behaviors are particularly troublesome to family members. Those cited most frequently include: physical violence and hitting, catastrophic reactions, suspiciousness and accusatory behavior, waking at night, and incontinence (Rabins et al, 1982). Certain suggestions are helpful in dealing with these behaviors.

Catastrophic reactions or excessive emotional reactions precipitated by task failure or minor stress can be minimized by teaching the family to avoid or remove the precipitating task or stress, to remain quiet and calm, and to gently change the focus of attention. Neuroleptics drugs are sometimes helpful but only as an adjunct to these techniques. Hitting and violent resistance to care are extreme catastrophic reactions and often can be eliminated or lessened in severity and frequency in these ways.

Caregivers frequently complain of chronic fatigue and when the patient awakens at night and wanders around the house, this further deprives the caregiver of much-needed rest. Certain environmental interventions are helpful. Locks can be placed on each door so that the patient will not wander out of the house at night and patients can be kept physically active during the day and not allowed to nap. Sedative-hypnotics, such as short-acting benzodiazepines or chloral hydrate, may be helpful. Occasionally, low doses of neuroleptics may be needed.

Suspiciousness and accusatory behaviors are serious problems which probably result from the brain-injured person's efforts to explain misplaced possessions or misinterpreted events. If the family understands this, their frustration, hurt, and anger may be reduced. Simple interventions, such as keeping an orderly house or making a sign pointing to where an object is kept, may help. Neuroleptics may be used as a last resort.

Incontinence is typically a late manifestation of Alzheimer's disease and when present early warrants a careful search for other causes, such as urinary tract infection.

Alzheimer's patients may decompensate cognitively and behaviorally when they experience a superimposed illness. Coexistent medical problems, such as asthma, diabetes, and congestive heart failure, should be carefully controlled. Even a minor upper respiratory tract or urinary tract infection can worsen behavior. Patients are susceptible to medication-induced delirium and close supervision of drug regimens is also imperative.

Family members can be reassured that inappropriate sexual behavior is very uncommon and in the rare instances where it occurs, self-stimulation is the usual form. Alzheimer's patients are not child molesters.

Not infrequently patients will want to drive when it is clear that they are no longer safe on the roads. If possible, it is best to avoid direct confrontation. Simple techniques such as hiding the keys, disconnecting distributor wires, or giving the patient a nonfunctional set of keys have usually been successful in discouraging patients from driving.

Firearms should not be kept in the home for obvious reasons. In addition, smoking and cooking become potentially dangerous activities. Environmental modifications, such as removing stove knobs, having a stove cut-off switch placed in an inconspicious place, locking rooms or closets, or locking up matches, are important for safety.

Family members report that lack of time for themselves and sleep disturbances in patients are the least tolerable aspects of home care. Studies have shown that "family support" was the major variable in keeping the cognitively impaired elderly at home. Families do best when relatives and friends visit frequently and when provisions are made for the primary caregiver to have breaks in his or her responsibilities. Visiting nurses or day-care centers can be invaluable.

SUMMARY

Alzheimer's disease is reaching epidemic proportions as the percentage of older Americans continues to rise. It is estimated that 20% of those over age 80 suffer from this illness and that half of all nursing home beds are filled by Alzheimer's patients. Because of these startling figures, all physicians will come into contact with these patients, both in their practices as well as in their personal lives.

The diagnosis is best made by looking at the overall course of the illness: slowly progressive decline; and by ruling out other causes of dementia. Every patient deserves a complete workup which has been outlined. Brain failure requires as thorough an evaluation as heart failure or renal failure. Many other illnesses, some treatable, can produce dementia. The dexamethasone suppression test (DST) may turn out to be a diagnostic aid which may help separate the pseudodementia of depression from the cognitive decline of *early* Alzheimer's disease. Advanced dementia alone (without overt depression) appears to produce an abnormal DST. Further work is required to clarify these issues.

The cause of Alzheimer's disease remains unknown. Four main theories have been discussed: genetic, viral, aluminum, and immune.

Once treatable causes for dementia have been eliminated, the primary care physician must manage a patient with a chronic and progressive illness. Physicians who prefer not to handle such patients should refer them to a colleague or geriatric specialist. Management necessitates that the physician assist family members, who may keep the patient at home until very late in the course of the illness, and be familiar with the use of psychotropic drugs. Many Alzheimer's victims will suffer concomitant depression, psychosis, anxiety, or behavior abnormalities which are generally responsive to medication. Tremendous research is now under way on specific drugs for memory enhancement. The finding that the cholinergic system is dramatically altered in Alzheimer's brains has suggested a large number of innovative approaches. Although small improvements in test scores can be achieved with some drugs, overall clinical improvement is unlikely. A six-month trial of Hydergine may be of some benefit. Chelation therapy has no proven benefit and is very expensive.

Management of the family is discussed in terms of optimizing the patient's care at home. It is recommended that those involved in the care of a demented patient join the Alzheimer's Disease and Related Disorders Association (ADRDA).

REFERENCES

Banen DM: An ergot preparation (hydergine) for relief of symptoms of cerebrovascular insuffiency. *J Am Geriatr Soc* 20:22–24, 1972.

Bartus RT, Dean RL, Beer R, et al: The cholinergic hypothesis of geriatric memory dysfunction. *Science* 217:408–416, 1982.

Bazo AJ: An ergot alkaloid preparation (hydergine) versus papaverine in treating common complaints of the aged: Double-blind study. *J Am Geriatr Soc* 21:63–71, 1973.

Behan PO, Behan WMH: Possible immunological factors in Alzheimer's disease, in Glen AIM, Whalley LJ (eds): *Alzheimer's Disease. Early Recognition of Potentially Reversible Deficits.* London. Churchill Livingstone, 1979, pp 33–35.

Behan PO, Feldman RG: Serum proteins, amyloid, and Alzheimer's disease. *J Am Geriatr Soc* 18:792–797, 1970.

Bruce ME, Fraser H: Amyloid plaques in the brains of mice infected with scrapie: Morphological variation and staining properties. *Neuropathol Appl Neurobiol* 1:189–202, 1975.

Burger PC, Vogel FS: The development of the pathologic changes of Alzheimer's disease and senile dementia in patients with Down's syndrome. *Am J Pathol* 73:457–476, 1973.

Carroll BJ, Feinberg M, Greden JF, et al: A specific laboratory test for the diagnosis of melancholia. *Arch Gen Psychiatry* 38:15–22, 1981.

Cook RH, Schneck SA, Clark DB: Twins with Alzheimer's disease. *Arch Neurol* 38:300–301, 1981.

Cook RH, Ward BE, Austin JH: Studies in aging of the brain. IV. Familial Alzheimer's disease: Relation to transmissible dementia aneuploidy and microtubular defects. *Neurology (NY)* 29:1402–1412, 1979.

Crapper DR Krishnan SS, Dalton AJ: Brain aluminum distribution in Alzheimer's disease and experimental neurofibrillary degeneration. *Science* 180:511–513, 1973.

Crapper DR, Krishnan SS, Quittkat S: Aluminum, neurofibrillary degeneration and Alzheimer's disease. *Brain* 99:67–80, 1976.

Crook T, Cohen G (eds): *Physicians' Handbook on Psychotherapeutic Drug Use in the Elderly.* New Canaan, Conn, Mark Powley Associates, Inc, 1981.

Cummings JL, Benson DF: *Dementia: A Clinical Approach.* Boston, Butterworth Publishers, 1983.

Davies P: Neurotransmitter-related symptoms in SDAT. *Brain Res* 171:319, 1979.

DeBoni U, Crapper DR: Paired helical filaments of the Alzheimer's type in cultured neurones. *Nature* 271:566–568, 1978.

Delaney JF: Spinal fluid aluminum levels in patients with Alzheimer's disease. *Ann Neurol* 5:581, 1979.

Ditch M, Kelly FJ, Resnick O: An ergot preparation (hydergine) in the treatment of cerebrovascular disorders in the geriatric patient: double-blind study. *J Am Geriatr Soc* 19:208–217, 1971.

Dunea G, Mahurkar SD, Mamdani B, et al: Role of aluminum in dialysis dementia. *Ann Intern Med* 88:502–504, 1978.

Gajdusek DC, Zigas V: Degenerative disease of the central nervous system in New Guinea: The epidemic occurrence of "kuru" in the native population. *N Engl J Med* 257:974–978, 1957.

Gerin J: Symptomatic treatment of cerebrovascular insuffiency with hydergine. *Curr Ther Res* 11:539–546, 1969.

Gibbs CJ Jr, Gajdusek DC: Subacute spongifo m virus encephalopathies: The transmissible virus dementias, in Katzman R, Terry RD, Bick KL (eds): *Alzheimer's Disease: Senile Dementia and Related Disorders.* New York, Raven Press, 1978, pp 559–577.

Glenner GG: Current knowledge of amyloid deposits as applied to senile plaques and congophilic angiopathy, in Katzman R, Terry RD, Bick KL (eds): *Alzheimer's Disease: Senile Dementia and Related Disorders.* New York, Raven Press, 1978, pp 493–501.

Goodnick P, Gershon S: Chemotherapy of cognitive disorders in geriatric subjects. *J Clin Psychiatry* 45:196–209, 1984.

Gottfries CG, Adolfsson R, Aquilonius SM, et al: Biochemical changes in dementia disorders of Alzheimer's type (AD/SDAT). *Neurobiol Aging* 4:261–271, 1983.

Goudsmit JAAP, White BJ, Weitkamp LR, et al: Familial Alzheimer's disease in two kindreds of the same geographic and ethnic origin. *J Neurol Sci* 49:79–89, 1981.

Greden JF, Carroll BJ: The dexamethasone suppression test as a diagnostic aid in catatonia. *Am J Psychiatry* 136:1199, 1979.

Haase GR: Diseases presenting as dementia, in Wells CE (ed): *Dementia*, ed 2. Philadelphia , FA Davis Co, 1977, pp 27–67.

Hachinski VC, Iliff LD, Zilhka E, et al: Cerebral blood flow in dementia. Arch *Neurol* 32:632–637, 1975.

Hachinski VC, Lassen NA, Marshall J: Multi-infarct dementia. A cause of mental deterioration in the elderly. *Lancet* 2:207–210, 1974.

Henschke PJ, Bell Da, Cape RDT: Alzheimer's disease and HLA. *Tissue Antigens* 12:132–135, 1978.

Heston LL: Alzheimer's disease, trisomy 21, and myeloproliferative disorders: Associations suggestng a genetic diathesis. *Science* 196:322–323, 1976.

Heston LL, Mastri AR, Anderson VE, et al: Dementia of the Alzheimer type: Clinical genetics, natural history and associated conditions. *Arch Gen Psychiatry* 38:1085–1090, 1981.

Hollister LE, Yesavage J: Ergoloid mesylates for senile dementia: Unanswered questions. *Ann Intern Med* 100:894–898, 1984.

Horita A: Neuropharmacology and aging, in Roberts J, Adelman RC, Cristafalo VJ (eds): *Pharmacological Intervention in the Aging Process.* New York, Plenum Press, 1978.

Hourrigan J, Klingsporn A, Clark WW, et al: Epidemiology of scrapie in the United States, in Prusiner SJ, Hadlow WJ (eds): *Slow Transmissible Diseases of the Nervous System.* New York, Academic Press, 1979.

Jarvik LF, Altshuler KZ, Kato T, et al: Organic brain syndrome and chromosone loss in aged twins. *Dis Nerv Syst* 32:159–169, 1971.

Jarvik LF, Ruth V, Matsuyama SS: Organic brain syndrome and aging: A six year follow-up of surviving twins. *Arch Gen Psychiatry* 37:280–286, 1980.

Jellinger J: Neuropathological agents and dementia. *Acta Neurol Belg* 76:83–102, 1976.

Jenike MA: Dexamethasone suppression test as an aid to diagnosing, treating, and following depression in the elderly. *Topics in Geriatrics* 1:13, 1981.

Jenike MA: Treatable dementias. *Topics in Geriatrics* 1:1–2, 1982a.

Jenike MA: Dexamethasone suppression: A biological marker of depression. *Drug Therapy* 12:203–212, 1982b.

Jenike MA: Dexamethasone suppression test as a clinical aid in elderly depressed patients. *J Am Geriatr Soc* 31:45–48, 1982c.

Jenike MA: The dexamethasone suppression test in the elderly: An update. *Clin Gerontologist* 2:3–11, 1983a.

Jenike MA: Drug treatment of depression. *Topics in Geriatrics* Sept. 1983b.

Jenike MA: Treating anxiety in elderly patients. *Geriatrics* 38:115–119, 1983c.

Jenike MA: Monoamine oxidase inhibitors in elderly depressed patients. *J Am Geriatr Soc* 32:571–575, 1984a.

Jenike MA: Chelation therapy. *Topics in Geriatrics* 3:11–12, 1984b.

Jenike MA: Management of Alzheimer's disease, in Goroll AH, May L, Mulley A (eds): *Primary Care Medicine*. Philadelphia, Pa, JB Lippincott Co, 1985a.

Jenike MA: Use of psychopharmacologic agents in the elderly, in Goroll AH, May L, Mulley A (eds): *Primary Care Medicine*. Philadelphia, Pa, JB Lippincott, 1985b.

Jenike MA: MAO inhibitors as treatment for depressed patients with primary degenerative dementia (Alzheimer's disease). *Am J Psychiatry* (in press) 1985c.

Jenike MA, Albert MS: The dexamethasone suppression test in patients with presenile and senile dementia of the Alzheimer's type. *J Am Geriatr Soc* 32:441–444, 1984.

Jennings WG: An ergot alkaloid preparation (hydergine) versus placebo for treatment of symptoms of cerebrovascular insufficiency: double-blind study. *J Am Geriatri Soc* 20:407–412, 1972.

Jonker C, Eikelenboom P, Tavenier P: Immunological indices in the cerebrospinal fluid of patients with presenile dementia of the Alzheimer's type. *Br J Psychiatry* 140:44–49, 1982.

Klatzo I, Wisniewski H, Streicher E: Experimental production of neurofibrillary degeneration. I. Light microscopic observations. *J Neuropathol Exp Neurol* 24:187–199, 1965.

Larsson T, Sjogren T, Jacobson G: Senile dementia. *Acta Psychiatr Scand* 39(suppl 167):3–259, 1963.

Lederman RJ, Henry CE: Progressive diaiysis encephalopathy. *Ann Neurol* 4:199–204, 1978.

Lishman WA: *Organic Psychiatry*. London, Blackwell Scientific Publications, 1978.

Mace NI, Rabins PV: *The 36-Hour Day*. Baltimore, The Johns Hopkins University Press, 1981.

Markesbery WR, Ehmann WD, Hossain TIM, et al: Brain trace element levels in Alzheimer's disease by instrumental neutron activation analysis. *J Neuropathol Exp Neurol* 40:359, 1981.

Marsh RF, Semancik JS, Medappa KC, et al: Scrapie and transmissible mink encephalopathy: Search for infectious nucleic acid. *J Virol* 13:993–996, 1974.

Mattis S: Dementia Rating Scale, in Bellack R, Karasu B (eds): *Geriatric Psychiatry*. New York, Grune & Stratton Inc, 1976.

McAllister TW, Ferrell RB, Price TRP, et al: The dexamethasone suppression test in two patients with severe depressive pseudodementia. *Am J Psychiatry* 139:479, 1982.

McConnachie RW: A clinical trial comparing "hydergine" with placebo in the treatment of cerebrovascular insuffiency in elderly patients. *Curr Med Res Opin* 1:463–468, 1973.

McDermott JR, Smith AI, Iqbal K, et al: Aluminum and Alzheimer's disease. *Lancet* 2:710–711, 1977.

McDermott JR, Smith AI, Iqbal K, et al: Brain aluminum in aging and Alzheimer's disease. *Neurology* 29:809-814, 1979.

Miller AE, Neighbor A, Katzman R, et al: Immunological studies in senile dementia of the Alzheimer's type: Evidence for enhanced suppressor cell activity. *Ann Neurol* 10:506-510, 1981.

Mortimer JA, Schuman LM (eds): *The Epidemiology of Dementia.* New York, Oxford University Press, 1981.

Nandy K: Brain-reactive antibodies in aging and senile dementia, in Katzman R, Terry RD, Bick KL (eds): *Alzheimer's Disease: Senile Dementia and Related Disorders.* New York, Raven Press, 1978, pp 503-512.

O'Daniel R, Lippmann S, Piyush P: Depressive pseudodementia. *Psychiatr Ann* 11:10-15, 1981.

Owens D, Dawson JC, Lowsin S: Alzheimer's disease in Down's syndrome. *Am J Ment Defic* 75:606-612, 1971.

Prusiner SD: Prions. *Sci Am* 251:50-59, 1984.

Rabins PV: Management of dementia in the family context. *Psychosomatics* 25:369-375, 1984.

Rabins PV, Mace NL, Lucas MJ: The impact of dementia on the family. *JAMA* 248:333-335, 1982.

Rao DB, Norris JR: A double-blind investigation of hydergine in the treatment of cerebrovascular insufficiency in the elderly. *Johns Hopkins Med J* 130:317-324, 1972.

Raskind M, Peskind E, Rivard MF, et al: Dexamethasone suppression test and cortisol circadian rhythm in primary degenerative dementia. *Am J Psychiatry* 139:1468, 1982.

Rehman SA: Two trials comparing "hydergine" with placebo in the treatment of patients suffering from cerebrovascular insufficiency. *Curr Med Res Opin* 1:456-462, 1973.

Reisberg B, Ferris SH, DeLeon MJ, et al: The Global Deterioration Scale for assessment of primary degenerative dementia. *Am J Psychiatry* 139:1136-1139, 1982.

Reisberg B, Ferris SH, Gershon S: An overview of pharmacologic treatment of cognitive decline in the aged. *Am J Psychiatry* 138:593-600, 1981.

Robinson DS: Changes in monoamine oxidase and monoamines with human development and aging. *Fed Proc* 34:103-107, 1975.

Robinson DS, David JM, Nies A, et al: Ageing, monoamines, and monoamine oxidase levels. *Lancet* 1:290-291, 1972.

Roos R, Gajdusek DC, Gibbs CJ: The clinical characteristics of transmissible Creutzfeldt-Jakob disease. *Brain* 96:1-20, 1973.

Rosen HJ: Mental decline in the elderly: Pharmacotherapy (ergot alkaloids versus papaverine). *J Am Geriatr Soc* 23:169-174 1975.

Roth M, Tomlinson BE, Blessed G: Correlation between scores for dementia and counts of "senile plaques" in grey matter of elderly subjects. *Nature* 209:109, 1966.

Roubicek J, Geiger C, Abt K: An ergot alkaloid preparation (hydergine) in geriatric therapy. *J Am Geriatr Soc* 20:222-229, 1972.

Rozas VV, Port FK, Rutt WM: Progressive dialysis encephalopathy from dialysate aluminum. *Arch Intern Med* 138:1375-1377, 1978.

Rudorfer MV, Clayton PJ: Depression, dementia, and dexamethasone suppression, letter. *Am J Psychiatry* 138:701, 1981.

Schlesser MA, Winokur G, Sherman BM: Hypothalamic-pituitary-adrenal axis activity in depressive illness: Its relationship to classification. *Arch Gen Psychiatry* 37:737, 1980.

Shore D, Millson M, Holtz JL, et al: Serum aluminum in primary degenerative dementia. *Biol Psychiatry* 15:971–977, 1980.

Sourander P, Sjogren H: The concept of Alzheimer's disease and its clinical implications, in Wolstenholme GEW, O'Connor M (eds): *Alzheimer's Disease and Related Conditions: A Ciba Foundation Symposium.* London, Churchill, 1970, pp 11–36.

Spar JE, Gerner R: Does the dexamethasone suppression test distinguish dementia from depression? *Am J Psychiatry* 139:238, 1982.

Spiegel R, Huber F, Koberle S: A controlled long-term study of ergoloid mesylates (hydergine) in healthy volunteers. *J Am Geriatr Soc* 31:549–555, 1983.

Sulkava R, Kiskimies S, Wikstrom J, et al: HLA antigens in Alzheimer's disease. *Tissue Antigens* 16:191–194, 1980.

Terry RD, Katzman R: Senile dementia of the Alzheimer type. *Ann Neurol* 14:497–506, 1983.

Terry RD, Pena C: Experimental production of neurofibrillary degeneration. II. Electron microscopy, phosphatase histochemistry and electron probe analysis. *J Neuropathol Exp Neurol* 24:200–210, 1965.

Thal L, Masur D, Fuld P, et al: Memory improvement with oral physostigmine and lecithin in Alzheimer's disease, in Katzman R (ed): *Banbury Report 15: Biological Aspects of Alzheimer's Disease.* New York, Cold Spring Harbor Laboratory, 1983, pp 461–469.

Thibault A: A double-blind evaluation of "hydergine" and placebo in the treatment of patients with organic brain syndrome and cerebral arteriosclerosis in a nursing home. *Curr Med Res Opin* 2:482–487, 1974.

Tomlinson BE, Blessed G, Roth M: Observations on the brains of non-demented old people. *J Neurol Sci* 7:331–356, 1968.

Tomlinson BE, Blessed G, Roth M: Observations on the brains of demented old people. *J Neurol Sci* 11:205–242, 1970.

Tourigny-Rivard MF, Raskind M, Rivard D: The dexamethasone suppression test in an elderly population. *Biol Psychiatry* 16:1177, 1981.

Triboletti F, Ferri H: Hydergine for treatment of symptoms of cerebrovascular insufficiency. *Curr Ther Res* 11:609–620, 1969.

Wells CE: Diagnostic evaluation and treatment in dementia, in Wells CE (ed): *Dementia*, ed 2. Philadelphia, FA Davis Co, 1977, pp 247–273.

Wells CE: Pseudodementia. *Am J Psychiatry* 136:895–900, 1979.

Wells CE: A deluge of dementia. *Psychosomatics* 22:836–840, 1981.

Whalley LJ, Urbaniak SJ, Darg C, et al: Histocompatibility antigens and antibodies to viral and other antigens in Alzheimer's presenile dementia. *Acta Psychiatr Scand* 61:1–7, 1980.

Wisniewski HM, Terry RD: Reexamination of the pathogenesis of the senile plaque, in Zimmerman HM (ed): *Progress in Neuropathology.* New York, Grune & Stratton Inc, 1973.

Wisniewski HM, Terry RD, Hirano A: Neurofibrillary pathology. *J Neuropathol Exp Neurol* 29:163–176, 1970.

Yates CM: Aluminum and Alzheimer's disease, in Glen AIM, Whalley LJ (eds): *Alzheimer's Disease. Early Recognition of Potentially Reversible Deficits.* London, Churchill Livingstone, 1979 pp 53–56.

CHAPTER 7

Insomnia

CHANGES IN SLEEP WITH INCREASING AGE

Difficulties with sleep are one of the most common complaints of elderly patients. Physicians should use medication only as a last resort to treat such difficulties.

With aging there are natural changes in sleep architecture which must be considered normal and are not altered significantly by medication. As infants we sleep most of the day; with increasing age the lengthy deep sleep of childhood naturally evolves into the lighter, shorter, and interrupted sleep of old age. As we age, we tend to spend more time in bed although actual sleep time tends to decline (Regestein, 1984). Sleep latency (the time it takes to get to sleep) lengthens, and sleep is normally interrupted by an increased number of awakenings (Miles and Dement, 1980). It is important that clinicians be aware of these *normal* changes with aging so that unnecessary drugs are avoided (Coleman et al, 1981; Greenblatt, 1978).

DRUGS AND ILLNESSES ASSOCIATED
WITH INSOMNIA

A number of drugs are clearly associated with altered sleep patterns. One of the most common offenders is caffeine (also found in tea and soft drinks as well as coffee), whose stimulant action may last well over 12 hours after a single cup of coffee in an elderly patient (Brezinova, 1974). In chronic alcohol abusers, sleep is uniformly impaired, both during abstinence and while drinking (Wagmen and Allen, 1975). Smoking is well documented as a cause of lighter sleep (Myrsten et al, 1977) and smokers obtain significantly improved sleep within a week after they stop (Regestein, 1984). Over-the-counter agents like cold tablets, nasal decongestants, stimulants, and appetite suppressants frequently interrupt sleep patterns of the elderly. Many prescription drugs, including antiarrhythmic agents, methysergide, thyroid hormones, steroids, methyldopa, epinephrine, and theophylline commonly produce some stimulation and may reduce sleep depth or onset.

Numerous medical illnesses are associated with sleep difficulty. Common offenders include arthritis or other pain-inducing diseases, restless-leg syndrome, itching, diabetes mellitus, hyperthyroidism, respiratory disease and sleep apnea, angina, and paroxysmal nocturnal dyspnea. Dementing illnesses such as Alzheimer's disease, multiinfarct dementia, parkinsonian dementia, and normal pressure hydrocephalus are associated with increased sleep difficulty.

Psychological causes of sleep difficulty are myriad — ranging from simple worries to severe endogenous depression. Sometimes boredom and lack of daytime stimulation lead to frequent naps during the day with resultant nighttime awakening. Many elderly patients go to bed at 7 or 8 PM and wake at 2 or 3 AM and do actually get enough sleep even though they may complain vigorously of insomnia. In all elderly patients complaining of insomnia, especially if early morning awakening is present, clinical depression should be sought by inquiring about the SIG E CAPS criteria (see chapter 4).

SLEEP RECORDS

Because of the variety of sleep difficulties, it is mandatory that the clinician carefully outline the patient's individual problem. Sleep logs are used commonly by sleep researchers. Patients are asked to document when they go to bed, when they fall asleep, the number and time of awakenings during the night, the time of morning awakening, and time of getting out of bed. This will aid the clinician in differentiating problems of sleep latency, interrupted sleep, or early morning awakening and will assist both diagnostically and therapeutically.

NONPHARMACOLOGIC TREATMENT
OF INSOMNIA

Medications should be avoided if at all possible. A number of simple manipulations may improve the quality of sleep in many patients (Table 7-1). If a patient is expecting that his/her sleep will not change with increasing age, education may be extremely beneficial. If interrupted lighter sleep can be redefined as normal, many elderly patients

Table 7-1
Nonpharmacologic Treatment of Insomnia

Education: The elderly sleep lighter, waken more often, and sleep fewer hours. This is *normal.*

Evening fluid restriction decreases nocturia.

Discourage daytime napping.

Exercise regularly when permissible: Avoid evening exercise.

Avoid caffeine, nicotine, and alcohol.

Avoid prescription drugs that are stimulatory or attempt to give them early in the day.

Optimally manage medical illnesses, especially heart and lung disease.

Control nighttime pain.

Recommend regular times for going to bed and arising.

Reproduced with permission from Jenike MA: Insomnia: Non-pharmacologic treatments. *Topics in Geriatrics* 3:25, 1984.

will seem relieved and be less concerned with forcing themselves to sleep. Once the pressure is off, some patients will be more relaxed and sleep quality will improve.

Daytime napping should generally be discouraged and activities should become part of the daily routine of all elderly patients, particularly those who are institutionalized. When it can be safely recommended, exercise is usually beneficial when done early in the day. Evening exercise may lead to increased arousal and difficulty getting to sleep.

Patients with severe insomnia should be advised to discontinue caffeine, alcohol, and cigarette smoking. Even one morning cup of coffee can contribute to nighttime sleep problems. Prescription medications should be adjusted so that nighttime stimulatory side effects are minimized.

Patients should set regular times for going to bed and for getting up in the morning. They should stay in bed a preset amount of time which should be based on the average daily amount of sleep time (Regestein, 1984).

Not infrequently the elderly awaken many times in the night to urinate. Urinary system problems should be evaluated and treated (eg, enlarged prostate). If no pathology is found, evening fluid restriction will decrease the frequency of nocturia.

Medical problems such as congestive heart failure, emphysema, and arthritis should be under optimal medical control to minimize night-time symptoms.

DRUG TREATMENT OF INSOMNIA

When sleep disturbances are severe and do not respond to non-pharmacologic approaches, a number of drugs may be helpful (Table 7-2). Neuroleptics (see chapter 3) and antidepressants (see chapter 4) should be avoided in nonpsychotic and nondepressed patients.

Many of the antianxiety agents (see chapter 5) are also helpful for treating insomnia. As when treating anxiety, it seems reasonable to avoid using the barbiturates and older agents such as meprobamate (Miltown) and ethchlorvynol (Placidyl) as first line agents. Tolerance develops rapidly to these agents and they are very addicting (Ewing and Bakewell, 1967; Kales et al, 1974).

Table 7-2
Drugs Used to Treat Insomnia

Drug	Dosage	Problems
L-Tryptophan	500 mg–2 g	None
Chloral Hydrate	500 mg–2 g	Gastric irritation Induces liver enzymes
Diphenhydramine	25–50 mg	Anticholinergic
Benzodiazepines		
Short-Acting		
Oxazepam	10–30 mg	
Lorazepam	0.5–2 mg	Amnesia very rare
Alprazolam	0.125–0.5 mg	Occasional daytime
Triazolam	0.25–0.5 mg	sedation
Temazepam	15–30 mg	
Long-Acting		
Flurazepam	15 mg	Active metabolites Very long-acting Daytime drowsiness, lethargy, ataxia
Sedating Antidepressants		
Trazodone	50–400 mg	Only when depressed
Nortriptyline	50–200 mg	

L-Tryptophan

L-Tryptophan is an amino acid which is metabolized to seroto-nin. Serotonin is felt to be involved in the regulation of deep sleep and has been shown to significantly reduce sleep latency in normal volunteers. It is probably worth trying in those elderly patients whose primary difficulty is falling asleep (Hartman et al, 1971; 1974; Bernstein, 1983). L-Tryptophan can be purchased as 500 mg tablets in most so-called health-food stores. Since it is not approved by the Food and Drug Administration, it is not available at this time in pharmacies. Initially, 500 mg should be prescribed at bedtime; this may be increased to as much as 2 g. L-Tryptophan, although relatively expensive, is very safe and should be tried initially if sleep latency difficulties are part of the clinical picture (Cole et al, 1980).

Chloral Hydrate

Chloral hydrate is a time-tested, safe medication which is very effective in the elderly. It exerts a rapid hypnotic effect and has a relatively short elimination half-life of approximately eight hours (Regestein, 1984). Drug interactions with chloral hydrate are uncommon (Greenblatt, 1981) and it is less likely to induce dependence and distort sleep patterns than the barbiturates and related drugs (Regestein, 1984). Its main drawbacks are that it sometimes produces gastrointestinal (GI) discomfort and excessive bowel flatus and that it induces hepatic enzymes increasing the rate of metabolism of other drugs such as the anticoagulants. Although doses of 500 mg are frequently effective, up to 2 g may be needed. It is supplied either as rather large 500-mg pills or as a syrup. It is one of the cheapest hypnotics available (Linnoila et al, 1980).

Antihistamines

Sedating antihistamines, such as diphenhydramine hydrochloride (Benadryl), are sometimes effective in speeding the onset of sleep in a patient with an otherwise relatively normal sleep pattern. Reportedly, tolerance to their sedative effects develops after several weeks (Regestein, 1984). At a dose of 25 to 50 mg given orally about a half-hour before bedtime, these agents are relatively safe. They do, however, have fairly potent anticholinergic effects and may on their own produce central or peripheral anticholinergic symptoms (see chapter 8). These effects are additive with other anticholinergic drugs. Because of the anticholinergic effects, these agents are probably not the best choice for patients with Alzheimer's disease because the cholinergic system is already not functioning optimally and even a mild anticholinergic load may precipitate clinical deterioration (see chapter 6). Antihistamines are the most common ingredient in over-the-counter sleep-inducing aids.

Benzodiazepines

Benzodiazepines are widely used as hypnotic agents and are considered to be very safe drugs in the elderly. The same considerations outlined in chapter 5 for use as antianxiety agents apply here. These drugs do not induce hepatic enzymes and are unlikely to be lethal on overdose when taken alone.

When long-acting agents, such as flurazepam (Dalmane), diazepam (Valium), or clorazepate (Tranxene), are used, there is a significant danger of a gradual build-up of long-acting metabolites with resulting daytime drowsiness and lethargy. Even though flurazepam is marketed as a hypnotic agent, it is apparently no better at inducing sleep than other benzodiazepines. It does, however, have one of the longest half-lives (Greenblatt et al, 1981) and when used in the elderly should be used briefly in low doses (15 mg) (Roth et al, 1979; 1980).

The short-acting benzodiazepines have fewer or no active metabolites and are rapidly eliminated. These shorter half-lives may be an advantage to older patients because the drugs are not likely to accumulate and produce daytime sedation (Merlis and Koepke, 1975). Benzodiazepines are not helpful in preventing early morning awakening and have even been reported to produce early morning insomnia when used continuously for a couple of weeks (Kales et al, 1983). For this reason, they should not be used on a daily basis for long periods. In addition, some of the short-acting agents have been reported to be associated with retrograde and anterograde amnesia (Regestein, 1984) (see chapter 5). Clinically, however, this must be very rare since a number of experienced geriatricians have never seen this. Lorazepam (Ativan) and oxazepam (Serax) have been around for many years and are generally very safe and effective for brief periods. These agents are relatively slowly absorbed and should be given about an hour prior to going to bed. Dosages range from 10 to 30 mg for oxazepam and from 0.5 to 2.0 mg for lorazepam. Triazolam (Halcion), temazepam (Restoril), and alprazolam (Xanax) are newer agents that may be as safe and effective as the older agents.

Alcohol

Small doses of alcohol are sometimes effective sleep aids. This may be best prescribed in carefully controlled environments such as nursing homes. Not all patients will respond and the dangers of dependence, addiction, and morning hangover are important (Regestein, 1984; Mishara and Kastenbaum, 1974; Stone, 1980).

SUMMARY

1. Carefully diagnose the specific problem. Difficulties are typically with sleep latency, interrupted sleep, or early morning awakening. Sleep logs may be helpful.
2. Normal elderly patients require less sleep and their sleep is typically lighter with more awakenings. Advising the patient of this is often therapeutic in and of itself.
3. A careful medical and drug history may illuminate potential causes of insomnia. Caffeine, nicotine, and alcohol should be temporarily discontinued. Discontinue offending drugs or adjust dosing schedule to minimize evening stimulation. Optimally control medical illnesses.
4. Carefully rule out depression. When depression is present, a sedating antidepressant is the most effective medication. Early morning awakening is very common with depression.
5. Avoid hypnotic medications initially and try to get the patient to avoid daytime naps and to get regular exercise when possible.
6. Advise patients to set regular times for going to bed and awakening.
7. If nocturia is a problem, rule out urinary system pathology and have patient avoid drinking fluids in the evening.
8. If nonpharmacologic approaches fail, a relatively brief trial of medication should be considered. L-Tryptophan is a reasonable, but relatively expensive, agent to try initially if the patient has trouble getting to sleep.
9. Chloral hydrate is safe and effective with minimal side effects.
10. Antihistamines can be prescribed and are common ingredients in over-the-counter preparations. They have anticholinergic effects which will be additive with other drugs.
11. Benzodiazepines are the most commonly used hypnotics. Long-acting agents have active metabolites and are best avoided in the elderly. Short-acting drugs, such as lorazepam and oxazepam, are

150

helpful for relatively short periods of time. Newer agents are available which may be as safe and effective.
12. Alcohol may be effective in some patients under carefully controlled situations.

REFERENCES

Bernstein JG: *Drug Therapy in Psychiatry*. Boston, Wright-PSG, 1983.

Brezinova V: Effect of caffeine on sleep: EEG study in late middle age. *Br J Clin Pharmacol* 1:203–208, 1974.

Cole JO, Hartmann E, Brigham P: L-tryptophan: Clinical studies. *McLean Hosp J* 5:37–71, 1980.

Coleman RM, Miles LE, Guilleminault C, et al: Sleep-wake disorders in the elderly: A polysomnograhic analysis. *J Am Geriatr Soc* 29:289–296, 1981.

Ewing JA, Bakewell WE: Diagnosis and management of depressant drug dependence. *Am J Psychiatry* 123:909–917, 1967.

Greenblatt DJ: Drug therapy of insomnia, in Rernstein JG (ed): *Clinical Psychopharmacology*. Littleton, Mass, PSG Publishing Co Inc, 1978, pp 27–39.

Greenblatt DJ: Sedative-hypnotics: Sleep disorders in the elderly, in Crook T, Cohen G (eds): *Physician's Handbook on Psychotherapeutic Drug Use in the Elderly*. New Canaan, Conn, Mark Powley Associates, Inc, 1981, pp 59–65.

Greenblatt DJ, Divoll M, Harmatz JS, et al: Kinetics and clinical effects of flurazepam in young and elderly insomniacs. *Clin Pharmacol Ther* 30:475–486, 1981.

Hartmann E, Chung R, Chien C: L-Tryptophan and sleep. *Psychopharmacologia* 19:114–127, 1971.

Hartmann E, Cravens J, List S: Hypnotic effects of L-Tryptophan. *Arch Gen Psychiatry* 31:394–397, 1974.

Kales A, Bixler EO, Tan TL, et al: Chronic hypnotic drug use. *JAMA* 227:513–517, 1974.

Kales A, Soldatos CR, Bixler EO, et al: Early morning insomnia with rapidly eliminated benzodiazepines. *Science* 220:95–97, 1983.

Linnoila M, Viukari M, Numminen A, et al: Efficacy and side effects of chloral hydrate and tryptophan as sleeping aids in psychogeriatric patients. *Pharmacopsychiatry* 15:124–128, 1980.

Merlis S, Koepke HH: The use of oxazepam in elderly patients. *Dis Nerv Syst* 36:27–29, 1975.

Miles LE, Dement WC: Sleep and aging. *Sleep* 3:119–220, 1980.

Mishara BL, Kastenbaum R: Wine in the treatment of long-term geriatric patients in mental institutions. *J Am Geriatr Soc* 22:88–94, 1974.

Myrsten AL, Elgerot A, Edgren B: Effects of abstinence from tobacco smoking on physiological and psychological arousal levels in habitual smokers. *Psychosom Med* 39:25–38, 1977.

Regestein QR: Treatment of insomnia in the elderly, in Salzman C (ed): *Clinical Geriatric Psychopharmacology*. New York, McGraw-Hill Book Co, 1984, pp 149–170.

Roth T, Hartze KM, Zorick FJ, et al: The differential effects of short- and long-acting benzodiazepines upon nocturnal sleep and daytime performance. *Drug Res* 30:891–894, 1980.

Roth T, Piccione P, Salis P, et al: Effects of temazepam, flurazepam, and quinalbarbitone on sleep: Psychomotor and cognitive function. *Br J Clin Pharmacol* 8:47S–54S, 1979.

Stone BM: Sleep and low doses of alcohol. *Electroencephalogr Clin Neurophysiol* 48:706–709, 1980.

Wagmen AM, Allen RP: Effects of alcohol ingestion and abstinence on slow wave sleep of alcoholics. *Adv Exp Med Biol* 59:453–466, 1975.

CHAPTER **8**

Anticholinergic Delirium:
Diagnosis and Treatment

Many of the drugs discussed in this book may be associated with anticholingeric side effects. Delirium is frequently induced in elderly patients by such agents. It is also well established that over 600 commonly used drugs have anticholinergic actions which can produce serious neuropsychiatric toxic effects (Granacher and Baldessarini, 1976). Diagnosis of delirium secondary to anticholinergic agents is tentatively established when there is a history of recent intake of one or more of these drugs, and when physical examination reveals the presence of peripheral muscarinic blockade. The latter may suggest the etiology of delirium when a history of drug exposure is uncertain or absent (Lipowski, 1980).

CLINICAL PICTURE

The signs and symptoms of peripheral muscarinic blockade include: dilated and poorly reactive pupils, tachycardia, facial flushing, dryness of skin and mucous membranes, blurred vision, urinary urgency, difficulty in initiating micturation, rise in blood pressure, and constipation. In some cases clinical manifestations such as fever, ataxia, dysarthria, muscle twitching, hyperreflexia, convulsions, and overactivity are present.

CLINICAL EXAMPLES

Case 1: A 73-year-old man was brought to the emergency room from a local nursing home after he became confused and agitated. About one week prior to this incident, he had been started on amitriptyline because of withdrawn behavior and depression. In addition to

153

confusion and agitation, the patient had a flushed face, dry skin, slight fever, and a pulse of 106. The physician diagnosed anticholinergic delirium and amitriptyline was discontinued.

Case 2: A 62-year-old woman had difficulty falling asleep for over a year. She treated herself with an over-the-counter medication which contained scopolamine. She gradually increased the dose to four capsules at bedtime. One night she awoke screaming. She was disoriented and convinced that her house was inhabited by strangers. Her husband took her to an emergency room where she was noted to have tachycardia and dilated pupils which were poorly responsive to light. She was treated with 1 mg physostigmine intramuscularly and her symptoms resolved.

COMMONLY IMPLICATED MEDICATONS

Nonprescription hypnotics Many of these contain small quantities of scopolamine. Sominex is a typical offender.

Cycloplegics and mydriatics Many elderly patients use eyedrops which contain atropine, scopolamine, and cyclopentolate. Even a small number of drops may induce delirium in the elderly. It is believed that such delirium may be due to swallowing of tears containing the drugs with subsequent absorption from the gastrointestinal (GI) tract. Eyedrops appear to be particularly likely to precipitate severe toxic-confusional reactions in the elderly or brain-damaged individual, and might lead to decompensation in mild dementia (Granacher and Baldessarini, 1976).

Antihistamines Drugs such as diphenhydramine (Benadryl), hydroxyzine (Vistaril, Atarax), and chlorpheniramine (Teldrin and others), and promethazine (Phenergan) are often prescribed as sedatives or antianxiety agents. These drugs have anticholinergic properties (Jenike, 1982a).

Anti-parkinsonian agents Benztropine (Cogentin), trihexyphenidyl (Artane), and procyclidine (Kemadrin) are frequently used in the treatment of both disease-related and drug-induced extrapyramidal motor disorders. As little as 2 mg of benztropine may produce delirium in some patients (Ananth and Jain, 1979).

Antipsychotic drugs Delirium with phenothiazine derivatives occurs most often in patients over age 50 and in brain-damaged patients (Angst and Hicklin, 1967; Helmchen, 1961). The delirium tends to follow rapid increases in dosage.

Low-potency neuroleptic drugs, such as chlorpromazine (Thorazine) and thioridazine (Mellaril), are much more likely to cause delirium than the high–potency drugs such as haloperidol (Haldol), fluphenazine (Prolixin), and thiothixene (Navane).

Antidepressants Tricyclic antidepressants are frequently associated with delirium in the elderly. Amitriptyline (Elavil and others) is the worse offender and has the highest antimuscarinic potency of the antidepressant drugs (see Table 8-1). Desipramine (Norpramin) has the least anticholinergic activity of the commonly used tricyclic antidepressants. Newer agents including maprotiline (Ludiomil) and trazodone (Desyrel) are said to have a low incidence of anticholinergic side effects (Gelenberg, 1981). Even in ordinary doses, antidepressants may produce a central delirium in the elderly without the striking peripheral parasympatholytic and pupillary signs seen with belladonna alkaloids (Baldessarini, 1978).

Other drugs Antispasmotic medications such as Lomotil, commonly used in GI disorders, frequently contain atropine sulfate. Cimetidine (Tagamet) has been reported to cause delirium in elderly patients (Jenike, 1982b). It is unclear at present if a central anticholinergic

Table 8-1
Antimuscarinic Potency of Commonly Used Drugs

Agent	Measure of Antimuscarinic Potency*
Scopolamine	0.3
Atropine	0.4
Trihexyphenidyl (Artane)	0.6
Benztropine (Cogentin)	1.5
Amitriptyline (Elavil)	10
Doxepin (Sinequan)	44
Imipramine (Tofranil)	78
Thioridazine (Mellaril)	150
Desipramine (Norpramin)	170
Chlorpromazine (Thorazine)	1000
Fluphenazine (Prolixin)	12,000
Thiothixene (Navane)	26,000
Haloperidol (Haldol)	48,000
Phenelzine (Nardil)	100,000

Adapted from Snyder et al (1974).
*The lower the number, the more likely the agent is to produce anticholinergic effects.

mechanism is responsible, but three cases have been reported where physostigmine rapidly reversed a presumed cimetidine-induced delirium (Mogelnicki et al, 1979; Jenike and Levy, 1983).

MANAGEMENT

If anticholinergic delirium is suspected, a trial of physostigmine (Antilirium) can be administered, typically by IM or *slow* IV injection in doses of 1 to 2 mg. If the patient's mental status improves and symptoms of muscarinic blockade resolve after physostigmine injection, the diagnosis is confirmed. Physostigmine, the only anticholinesterase to freely cross the blood-brain barrier and reverse central anticholinergic effects, inhibits cholinesterase and thus promotes the action of acetylcholine.

The use of physostigmine is not without complications, including precipitation of asthmatic episodes and heart block resulting in myocardial infarction (Hall et al, 1981). The most serious consequences of excessive or too rapid administration of physostigmine are the provocation of acute respiratory embarrassment, heart block, or seizure (Granacher and Baldessarini, 1976). Because of these and other possible complications, some clinicians feel that it should be used conservatively (Baldessarini and Gelenberg, 1979). One report, however, contained 1727 cases of successful treatment of central anticholinergic intoxication with no untoward effects (Holzgrafe et al, 1973). Toxicity due to physostigmine, manifested most commonly by nausea, vomiting, diarrhea, and bradycardia, may be reversed by the administration of 0.5 mg atropine sulfate for each milligram of physostigmine administered.

Physostigmine has a relatively short half-life of 90 to 120 minutes. Thus, when anticholinergic toxicity is secondary to long-acting drugs, physostigmine may be needed at intervals of 30 minutes to two hours. For a mild anticholinergic syndrome or in elderly confused patients with uncertain cardiac status, one can manage the patient by withdrawal of the suspected toxin and the use of protective measures, reassurance, plus a benzodiazepine, such as lorazepam (Ativan) or oxazepam (Serax). Other central depressants, which themselves have anticholinergic properties, should not be used (Granacher and Baldessarini, 1976).

SUMMARY

The elderly are particularly likely to develop an anticholinergic delirium. The diagnosis is made when a patient has recently taken a drug which is known to induce anticholinergic effects and when peripheral signs of anticholinergic toxicity are present.

Some of the commonly implicated agents include: nonprescription hypnotics, cycloplegics and mydriatics, antihistamines, antiparkinsonian agents, antipsychotic drugs, and antidepressants.

The management of delirious patients involves primarily withdrawal of the offending agent and, if symptoms are severe, the administration of physostigmine. Physostigmine has some inherent dangers, such as induction of acute respiratory problems, heart block, or seizure. These can generally be avoided if the drug is given intramuscularly or *slowly* intravenously. For mild cases, reassurance plus a benzodiazepine may be adequate treatment.

REFERENCES

Ananth JV, Jain RC: Benztropine psychosis. *Can J Psychiatry* 18:409–414, 1979.

Angst J, Hicklin A: Deliröse Psychosen unter Neuroleptica und Antidepressiva. *Schweiz Med Wochenschr* 97:546–549, 1967.

Baldessarini RJ: *Chemotherapy in Psychiatry.* Cambridge, Mass, Harvard University Press, 1978.

Baldessarini RJ, Gelenberg AJ: Using physostigmine safely. *Am J Psychiatry* 136:1609–1610, 1979.

Gelenberg AJ: New antidepressants. *Biol Ther Psychiatry* 4:5, 1981.

Granacher RP, Baldessarini RJ: The usefulness of physostigmine in neurology and psychiatry, in Klawans HL (ed): *Clinical Neuropharmacology.* New York, Raven Press, 1976, vol 1.

Hall RCW, Feinsilver DL, Holt RE: Anticholinergic psychosis: Diagnosis and treatment. *Psychosomatics* 22:581–587, 1981.

Helmchen H: Delirante Abläufe unter psychiatrischer Pharmakotherapie. *Arch Psychiatr Nervenkr* 202:395–411, 1961.

Holzgrafe RE, Vondrell JJ, Mintz SM: Reversal of postoperative reactions to scopolamine with physostigmine. *Anesth Analg (Cleve)* 52:921–925 1973.

Jenike MA: Using sedative drugs in the elderly. *Drug Therapy* 12:184–190, 1982a.

Jenike MA: Cimetidine in elderly patients: Review of uses and risks. *J Am Geriatr Soc* 30:170–173, 1982b.

Jenike MA, Levy JC: Physostigmine reversal of cimetidine-induced delirium and agitation. *J Clin Psychopharmacol* 3:43–44, 1983.

Lipowski ZJ: *Delirium.* Springfield, Ill., Charles C. Thomas, 1980.

Mogelnicki SR, Waller JL, Finlayson DC: Physostigmine reversal of cimetidine-induced mental confusion. *JAMA* 241:826–827, 1979.

Snyder S, Greenberg D, Yamamura H: Antimuscarinic potency of CNS agents. *Arch Gen Psychiatry* 31:173, 1974.

162